Health Care Matters

Health Care Matters

Pharmaceuticals, Obesity, and the Quality of Life

Richard D. Miller Jr.
and
H. E. Frech III

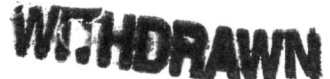

The AEI Press

Publisher for the American Enterprise Institute

WASHINGTON, D.C.

2004

Available in the United States from the AEI Press, c/o Client Distribution Services, 193 Edwards Drive, Jackson, TN 38301. To order, call toll free: 1-800-343-4499. Distributed outside the United States by arrangement with Eurospan, 3 Henrietta Street, London WC2E 8LU, England.

b# 221731

Library of Congress Cataloging-in-Publication Data
Miller, Richard D., Jr.
      Health care matters: pharmaceuticals, obesity, and the quality of life/
    Richard D. Miller Jr. and H. E. Frech III
          p. cm.
      Includes bibliographical references and index.
      ISBN 0-8447-4194-9 (pbk.)
      1. Pharmaceutical policy. 2. Health status indicators. 3. Obesity.
    4. Medical economics.
    I. Frech, H. E., III. II. Title.

    RA401.A1M557 2004
    362.17'82—dc22

                                                                    2003063646

1 3 5 7 9 10 8 6 4 2

Printed in the United States of America

Contents

Illustrations

Acknowledgments

Earlier versions of this work were presented in seminars at Curtin University in Perth, Australia, on June 21, 2001, and at the International Health Economics Association meetings in York, England, on July 24, 2001. Thanks are due to the participants of those seminars, especially Harry Bloch, Gavin Mooney, Jeff Petchy, and Sandra Hopkins. This work extends our earlier research, which was supported by a grant from Sciences Po de Paris. We are grateful for support for this research from Pfizer, Merck, AztraZeneca, and Bristol Myers-Squibb. Thanks are due to Dominic Esposito for excellent research assistance.

1

Introduction

For many years, health policy in wealthy countries has rested on the assumption that health-care consumption is not productive, that it does relatively little to produce better health. Researchers comparing health consumption from country to country have largely failed to find a relationship between it and actual health outcomes. This study shows that it is time to rethink this conventional wisdom, in particular as it relates to pharmaceutical consumption.

Greater pharmaceutical consumption leads not just to longer lives, but also to a higher quality of life, as measured by the number of years people can expect to live without disabling health conditions. In this study, which takes advantage of newly available data, we find that greater pharmaceutical use has an even stronger effect on the quality of life than it does on life expectancy. More specifically, we find that a 10 percent increase in pharmaceutical consumption would increase a sixty-year-old's disability-adjusted life expectancy (our measure of quality of life) by about 0.9 percent, and would raise his or her unadjusted life expectancy by 0.6 percent. We also find that our improved model and newer data reveal the relationship between pharmaceutical consumption and life expectancy to be even stronger than the relationship we uncovered in our previous research (Frech and Miller 1999; Miller and Frech 2000).

Greater pharmaceutical consumption strikes against mortality from circulatory disease, cancer, and respiratory disease—the ailments that together account for three out of four deaths in the wealthy countries of the Organisation for Economic Co-operation and Development (OECD). Greater drug use shows especially marked success in fighting circulatory disease, which alone accounts for four out of every ten deaths in OECD

1

countries. Specifically, a 10 percent increase in pharmaceutical consumption would decrease premature mortality (before the age of seventy) from circulatory disease by almost 2 percent. It would lower mortality for those ages sixty-five to seventy-four by about 3.6 percent, and for those ages seventy-five and over by 1.5 percent. Greater pharmaceutical use has far less effect on mortality due to cancer and respiratory disease, although it does lower cancer mortality among those over the age of seventy-five and respiratory disease mortality among those ages sixty-five to seventy-four.

In this study, we also estimate how much it would cost to raise life expectancy (or disability-adjusted life expectancy) with increased pharmaceutical consumption. Greater pharmaceutical consumption could greatly benefit society, being a relatively cheap way to extend life and improve health. In general, countries that currently spend the least on pharmaceuticals would see the greatest benefits from an increase in that spending.

However, our models tell us little about the relationship between consumption of nonpharmaceutical medical care and either quality of life or life expectancy. Likewise, the data tell us little about what effect nonpharmaceutical health-care consumption has on mortality due to the specific diseases we study here. When we do observe an effect, we are unable to form a clear conclusion as to its cause. Because consumption of nonpharmaceutical health-care services is so closely related to wealth in OECD countries, it is simply impossible to discern whether the observed effect is the result of spending more on health care or of being wealthier. In our previous research, we found no link between nonpharmaceutical health-care consumption and life expectancy.

Starting with the very basic assumption that an individual's health can be explained by his or her personal behavior, social status (wealth), and consumption of health-care goods and services (including pharmaceuticals), we can try to estimate how better health might be produced for a whole population, and at what cost.

To say the least, this endeavor raises many questions that continue to dog researchers in the field of health-care economics. For instance, how do we define health? Until recently, the only consistent way to do so—at least for the purpose of making comparisons across countries—was to define it as longer life expectancy or lower infant mortality. While both these measures are clearly important, they are hardly perfect for measuring the results of health-care consumption. In today's wealthy countries, consumption of health care and pharmaceuticals is intended not merely to increase survival at the beginning of life or longevity at the end. Rather, it aims to enable people to live fuller lives throughout the course of life, to improve the *quality* of their lives (Cutler and Richardson 1997). Heart surgery might add years to life while hip replacement surgery might not, but the latter enables many to have active lives free of pain. While a certain cancer drug might prolong survival, a medication for asthma might simply allow a person to exercise. Measuring improvement in the quality of life is a difficult exercise, especially when we try to compare it in different countries. Here, our research benefits directly from the recent work of the World Health Organization (WHO), which now produces data specifically for this purpose.

However, it is not just the limitations of available data that make assessing the productivity of health spending a complex task. Obviously, many factors combine to produce health. At a very basic level, public health measures such as the provision of clean drinking water and sanitation systems have a huge impact. Education and wealth can play a role. Lifestyle decisions, such as whether to smoke or how much to weigh, also play an increasingly important role in the health of the citizens of wealthy countries.

In our study, we analyze the effects of pharmaceutical and other health-care consumption in most of the OECD countries on health, life expectancy, and mortality due to circulatory diseases, cancer, and respiratory diseases. We also analyze the effects of wealth and three major lifestyle variables—smoking, drinking, and obesity—on those measures of health.

In most cases, we find that obesity outranks both smoking and drinking as a risk factor for health and life expectancy. Furthermore, obesity is a powerful predictor of circulatory disease, the most common cause of death in OECD countries. For cancer, the second most common cause of death, tobacco and alcohol consumption tend to have a greater effect than obesity, though it still plays a role. This research should draw further attention to obesity as a threat to public health.

The fact that pharmaceutical consumption produces better health has several important public policy implications. For one, it lends support to proposals to increase coverage of drugs in both public and private health insurance systems, especially for the elderly. That said, lurking behind many proposals to do this, with respect to public sector programs such as Medicare, is the impetus to control drug prices. An effort of this sort might well undermine the intended benefits. For instance, such a policy may decrease the costs faced by these public programs, but it is also likely that price controls would discourage the development of new drugs by lowering the potential return of drug research to drug manufacturers.

Most fundamentally, this study shows that policymakers should no longer base their proposals on the assumption that health-care consumption does not improve health, but rather on a new understanding that such consumption—especially pharmaceutical use—does matter.

2

Literature Review

To date, most researchers have compared health-care spending across different countries in order to study its determinants—how much is spent and what it is spent on.[1] Clearly, this approach has reflected a long-standing concern on the part of policymakers that burgeoning real spending threatened public-sector budgets and would continue to do so as the populations of wealthy countries began to age, and as ever more technologically advanced (and expensive) medical treatments became available.

Far fewer have compared health-care consumption across countries with the aim of determining whether it is productive—that is, whether it produces better health and does so in an economical way. As we have already mentioned, much of the existing literature, produced by scholars in a variety of disciplines often outside economics, has suggested that health-care consumption is fairly unproductive in the quest for better health.

The following sections will review our own previous research as well as other relevant studies, summarizing their main conclusions and discussing their methodologies. We believe it important to discuss these methodologies and data sources carefully, because they have often led researchers to faulty conclusions.

Conclusions from Our Earlier Literature Review

Studies of developing countries have shown increased medical consumption to have a much smaller effect on health than investments in such basic infrastructure as clean water and sanitation systems—the two most powerful factors in improving health in these countries. This conclusion strikes us as robust and sensible. Raising per-capita income and education levels has also been shown to be more powerful in improving health than raising actual health-care consumption in developing countries. The small impact of medical care in these studies has supported the conventional wisdom in health economics that it does little to improve life expectancy. But a few good studies have found medical care to matter, including a closely related one using OECD data (Zweifel and Ferrari 1992).

The closest precursor to our earlier study (see Frech and Miller 1999; Miller and Frech 2000) was by Akira Babazono and Alan Hillman (1994). Unusual for its time, it disaggregated health care to examine effects on perinatal and infant mortality and life expectancy. In contrast to our study, this one found no effect of pharmaceutical consumption on health measures.

However, Babazono and Hillman reached their conclusions after making several methodological errors. First, they used an overall purchasing power parity exchange rate to convert drug prices to common terms. When a certain drug costs $100 in the United States, $132 in Canada, and 1,090 yen in Japan, how should researchers convert these prices to common terms so that they can be compared to one another? Babazono and Hillman assumed that drug prices differed from country to country in the same way as prices for all other goods did.

As the current U.S. debate over relative drug prices in the United States and Canada shows, this is a seriously problematic assumption. More recently, Anders Anell and Michael Willis (2000, 772) made the same mistake, justifying it by arguing that there is a world market in pharmaceuticals. While this is true, most countries control the prices of drugs in one way or another, resulting in real differences across countries that must be accounted for when converting prices to common terms. We discuss this issue in greater detail in the section summarizing our own previous research.

The Babazono and Hillman research also suffered from incorrect functional form: The authors assumed there should be a linear relationship between health-care consumption and health—in other words, raising real health-care spending from $1,000 to $2,000 should have the same effect as raising it from $0 to $1,000. To an economist, this common assumption fails to account for diminishing marginal returns to health-care consumption. In the real world, the first $1,000 of health-care use should have a far more powerful effect on health than the next thousand, and so on.

Both of these assumptions are critical to modeling the production of health. Incorrect conversion of drug prices means the measure of actual drug consumption will be inaccurate. Failure to account for the diminishing marginal returns of health-care consumption makes it easy to misinterpret the results of a given model.

Our Earlier Work

Our own previous research on this subject remains the most relevant literature for this study. In the earlier work, our main finding was that pharmaceutical consumption has a surprisingly powerful impact on life expectancy of adults at ages forty and sixty. We found that a doubling of pharmaceutical use would increase life expectancy at age forty by about 2 percent and at age sixty by about 4 percent, a result that was both statistically and economically significant.

We showed, for each country, how much additional consumption of pharmaceuticals it would take to prolong life for one year. In high-pharmaceutical-consumption countries, the cost of saving a life year by additional consumption was much higher than in low-consumption countries. The estimates (in 1990 dollars, for males) ranged from $3,800 in Turkey to $60,000 in France. In the United States, a middling country in pharmaceutical consumption, the cost of saving a life year was $21,000. This was well below the value of a life year typically assumed by economists for policymaking purposes.

We obtained very similar results when we controlled for additional variables, such as population over sixty-five, unemployment, income inequality, or educational level, or excluded the lifestyle variables. Further, the results were not sensitive either to dropping Turkey (an outlier) or dropping all non-European observations.

We were unable to form clear conclusions about the effects of pharmaceutical consumption on infant mortality. Signs and magnitudes of effects were very sensitive to variations in specification that were small and easily defended. However, the lack of clear conclusions in this analysis may simply have revealed that infant mortality was a poor measure of health. The data on life expectancy at birth had similar shortcomings.

Our results also indicated no measurable effect on life expectancy at any age of nonpharmaceutical health consumption, and unclear effects on infant mortality. Gross domestic product (GDP), on the other hand, had positive and statistically significant effects on life expectancy, larger at more advanced ages.

The lifestyle variable with the biggest effect was fat consumption. At low levels, more fat consumption increased life expectancy, but at high levels it reduced it. This was fairly surprising. One might have thought that the OECD countries were all wealthy enough that nutrition, in terms of underconsumption, would not have been an issue

In this earlier analysis, we measured health by several crude but objectively observable variables: by life expectancy at birth, age forty, and age sixty; and by infant mortality. We used 1993 OECD life expectancy and infant mortality data from twenty-one countries as of the early 1990s, and we converted pharmaceutical and nonpharmaceutical health-care expenditures to U.S. dollars by using purchasing power parity (PPP) exchange rates specifically for pharmaceutical and all health-care expenditures, thus generating measures of real consumption.

The pharmaceutical PPP exchange rates were imperfect; but extensive analysis showed them to be by far the best available for more than a handful of countries, and we sought to avoid the methodological error made in earlier studies of measuring pharmaceutical consumption by using the wrong exchange rate. When we tested our own data with the incorrect rate, our results changed, showing the importance of using the correct one.

We used multivariate regressions to estimate production relationships, employing a specification that allowed for diminishing marginal returns to each input. Aside from the health-care variables discussed above, the regressions included GDP and several lifestyle variables: tobacco and alcohol consumption and the fat content of diet. These explanatory variable measures were from the 1983 to 1985 time period. Thus, we showed what effect they had on a population's life expectancy or infant mortality eight to ten years later.

Recent Aggregate Studies of the Production of Health

In this section, we summarize several more recent studies on the production of health. Like our research, these studies have begun to reveal that, in general, health-care consumption does help improve health.

Studies within the United States. In a unique study, Frank Lichtenberg (2000a) examined what effects U.S. health-care spending and Federal Drug Administration (FDA) new drug approvals had, several years later, on life expectancy at birth over the 1960 to 1997 time period. He studied the effects of both public and private health expenditures (but not pharmaceutical versus other expenditures) on whites, blacks, and the combined population. Lichtenberg found that health-care spending and new drug approvals had large positive and statistically significant effects on life expectancy at birth. His results indicate that doubling health-care spending would increase life expectancy by 7 percent. This is more than double the effect that we had found.

Lichtenberg found the marginal cost of saving one life year with health-care expenditures to be quite low, about $11,000. Assuming it cost about $500 million to get FDA approval for a new drug, a commonly cited figure, Lichtenberg calculated that it cost a very low $1,345 to save one life year through pharmaceutical innovation. Compared to what many authors have assumed to be the value of a life year—$150,000—both more health-care spending and more drug approvals scored extremely well. This research would also score well in terms of the marginal cost to save a life year.[2]

Lichtenberg interpreted the finding on new drug approvals as representing (or perhaps embodying) technical progress in health care in general. If one views technical progress as resulting entirely from medical R & D spending, rather than learning-by-doing and exogenous innovation from other scientific research (for example, basic chemistry), this roughly triples the cost per life year saved. But medical R & D is still a great bargain if one can take the estimates literally.

International Studies. In a cross-country study similar to ours, Zeynep Or (2000a, 2000b) also found health-care spending to have a large effect on health.

Using a sample of twenty-one OECD countries, spanning 1970 to 1992, Or (2000a) examined the effects of health-care spending (from OECD data) and other variables on premature mortality, or potential years of life lost (PYLL), calculated from unpublished mortality statistics from the WHO. Suicide was excluded.

Separate regressions were run for men and women. The model included variables for health-care spending, the share of that spending that was public, GDP, and lifestyle and environmental variables. A novel inclusion was a variable for the proportion of workers in white-collar jobs, which was intended to measure social status and education. The primary method used was ordinary least squares (OLS) with fixed effects, with dummy variables for each country. Or used a specification that was similar to the one that we used in our previous study described above. This specification allowed for diminishing returns in the production of health. Or found large effects of both medical consumption and GDP on premature mortality, especially for women. She found that doubling aggregate medical consumption would lower premature mortality by 18 percent for women and by nearly 4 percent for men. The estimate for women was statistically significant at high levels, while for men it was statistically weak. It is difficult to compare Or's work directly with ours because life expectancies and PYLL are not exactly inverses, even though both are expressed as years. Further, we disaggregated types of health-care consumption. Still, it is safe to say that Or found a much greater effect of health-care consumption on health for women than we did, and a comparable effect on men. The proportion of public spending was also important.

The proportion of workers in white-collar jobs was very important, as doubling this proportion would lower premature mortality by 81 percent for women and by 74 percent for men. Both results are highly significant. Or interpreted this as an environmental variable in the sense that it measures the social and intellectual environment of an individual. We believe it also reveals the effects of real income on health, by picking up some aspects of wealth not measured by GDP, such as a pleasant and safe workplace. (In a later paper discussed below, Or [2000b] showed that the simple correlation between GDP and the proportion of white-collar workers was very high, 0.8393.) Per-capita GDP had about half the effect of white-collar work, though it was also highly significant. Lifestyle variables and a variable for air pollution also had the expected effects on premature mortality. Country dummy variables were very important.

In a later paper, Or (2000b) expanded her reach. Instead of measuring health care with spending, she examined the effects of the doctor-to-population ratio on life expectancy at age sixty-five, premature mortality (PYLL) due to cancer, and heart disease, as well as perinatal and infant mortality. Further, she entered some variables to account for type of health-care system (for example, fee-for-service versus global budgeting for hospitals). She used a slightly shorter panel and a different econometric technique (feasible generalized least squares) to account for heteroskedasticity and serial correlation.[3]

The results of this second study were generally consistent with Or's earlier one, but they showed even larger effects of the doctor-to-population ratio than health spending. The results indicated that doubling the ratio would decrease premature mortality by 38 percent for women and by 28 percent for men. Note that the result for men was much stronger than in Or's previous study. The effect on infant and perinatal mortality was even higher, as was the effect on PYLL due to heart disease, while the effect on cancer was smaller. All of these results, except for male PYLL due to cancer, were statistically significant at a high level. The results for the type of system were weak and not robust. Sensitivity analyses, comparing this econometric method to fixed effects, showed generally similar results.

Because this study also examined life expectancy at age sixty-five, we can compare Or's results with ours. She found that doubling the doctor-to-population ratio would increase life expectancy at age sixty-five by 10 percent for both men and women. This is a much smaller effect than the ratio's effect on premature mortality, but it is still slightly more than twice as large as the effect of pharmaceutical consumption on life expectancy at sixty that we found in our previous research.

Or offered several sensible interpretations for the strong effects of the doctor-to-population ratio on health. Most convincing to us is the idea that higher doctor-to-population ratios are correlated with greater use of high-tech medicine. This is similar in principle to Lichtenberg's (2000a) interpretation of new drug approvals in the United States as having been the outcome of general medical research.

We can rule out the idea that measuring the use of high-tech medical equipment is a good way to reveal the effects of medical research. Perhaps surprisingly, the doctor-to-population ratio among rich countries is not strongly related to the use of such equipment. For example, on a per-capita basis, the United States had seven times as many MRI machines as France did in 1996. In 1991, the United States had almost four times as many CT scanners, yet the United States had fewer doctors (Anell and Willis 2000, 773).

We suspect that the doctor-to-population ratio is highly correlated with pharmaceutical consumption, however, and many pharmaceuticals embody the results of recent research. Explicit consideration of pharmaceutical consumption would be very interesting, but it cannot be done for more than a very small number of years, due to the lack of data on pharmaceutical purchasing parity exchange rates.

Or's results, as well as the results of the Lichtenberg studies discussed earlier, showed medical spending to be far more productive than most studies comparing spending across countries or regions have indicated. In both Or's and Lichtenberg's studies, the results were similar using country (but not time) fixed effects. This suggests that most of the explanatory power was coming from time-series variation. While the econometric problems of this approach are not fully worked out for panel data, this in turn suggests possible unit root problems with trended data, leading to spurious results. Studies focusing on the determinants of health-care spending have generally found unit roots in both GDP and health expenditures in both country-by-country and panel data (Hansen and King 1996, 1998; Bloomqvist and Carter 1997; Gerdtham and Lothgren 2000; MacDonald and Hopkins 2002). We would expect the same for life expectancy, since it is strongly trended. Unit roots may lead to spurious regression results (Pindyck and Rubinfeld 1998, 508–16; Hamilton 1994, 557–62; Kennedy 1998, 268–70). In other words, unit roots are a problem because they can cause bias in regression models. When unit roots are present, researchers may find relationships among variables when those relationships do not actually exist. Further, A. G. Bloomqvist and R. A. L. Carter (1997, 221, 225–26) have argued that, in this context, OLS is asymptotically biased and inefficient, and that the data strongly reject the pooling assumption, even with country fixed effects included. Thus, the strong results of both Or and Lichtenberg may have been overstated.

Epidemiological Studies of Risk Factors

Another way to look at how health is produced, at least with reference to some factors known to cause health problems, is by means of an epidemiological technique. Murray and Lopez (1997c, 1999) have analyzed the effects of certain risk factors in this way, using disability-adjusted life years (DALYs) as their measure of health. According to their analyses, the most significant risk factors were tobacco use (costing 11.7 percent of DALYs), followed by alcohol use (10.3 percent), occupation (5.0 percent), physical inactivity (4.8 percent), and hypertension (3.9 percent). Interestingly, air pollution ranked eighth, responsible for only 0.5 percent of DALYs (Murray and Lopez 1997c, 1440).

Note that physical inactivity and hypertension were related to obesity. This is convenient from an analytical standpoint because objective measures of obesity are available, both in time-series and cross-section. It may be possible to capture much of the variation in these two risk factors by including obesity in a statistical analysis.

While interesting, this epidemiological method, called attributable burden (Murray and Lopez 1999; 1997c, 1436–37), can be crude and subjective. It is based on the opinions of experts in various fields, which are, in turn, based at least partly on epidemiological studies of specific risk factors. The attributable burden is defined as the difference in burden between what is observed and what would occur with some specified reference exposure to the risk factor. In other words, it is the difference between, say, actual life expectancy in the United States and life expectancy if no Americans smoked. (Theoretically, the reference exposure could be anything, including zero. Murray and Lopez did not use zero, but rather some lower level that was viewed as somehow attainable.)

Attributable burden assumes that the risk factors can be distinguished from one another, and that they affect health in an additive fashion, without interacting with one another. It also assumes that the production function is a step function, where the extent of exposure doesn't matter, but only whether there is exposure or not. While the method is subjective, it allows analysts to summarize the information crudely in many different small-scale studies and surveys. The results are, at the least, suggestive for those estimating health production relations using ordinary statistical techniques.

Obesity

Obesity is a particularly interesting risk factor, because it is now on the rise in many countries. Among the rich countries, the United States has the highest obesity rates and, up until a few years ago, was in a class by itself. Today other countries, such as the United Kingdom and Australia, are catching up quickly. There is surprisingly large variation in obesity rates, even among the rich countries.

A person is typically considered obese if his or her body mass index (BMI) is thirty or higher. The BMI is simply the ratio of an individual's weight in kilograms to the square of that individual's height in meters. For example, a BMI of thirty corresponds to a person five feet, five inches tall, weighing 180 pounds (1.65 meters, 81.65 kilograms), or to a person five feet, ten inches tall, weighing 207 pounds (1.77 meters, 93.89 kilograms). Overweight is similarly defined as a BMI of over twenty-five, corresponding to 173 pounds for the five foot, ten inch person.

Both the level and the growth in obesity rates are impressive (see figure 1). For example, in 1999, 26 percent of United States adults were obese, up from 14.5 percent in 1978–80. In the United Kingdom, the obesity rate was 21 percent in 2000, up from only 7 percent in 1980. In Australia, it was 20.8 percent in 1999, up from 7.1 percent in 1980. At the other end of the scale (no pun intended), only 2.9 percent of Japanese adults were obese in 2000, up from 2 percent in 1980 (OECD 2003). Even in poor countries, obesity is becoming a major problem (Winslow and Landers 2002; Hill and Peters 1998). J. Michael McGinnis and William Foege (1993) used epidemiological methods to estimate that obesity causes 14 percent of

Figure 1: Adult Obesity, circa 1980 and circa 2000

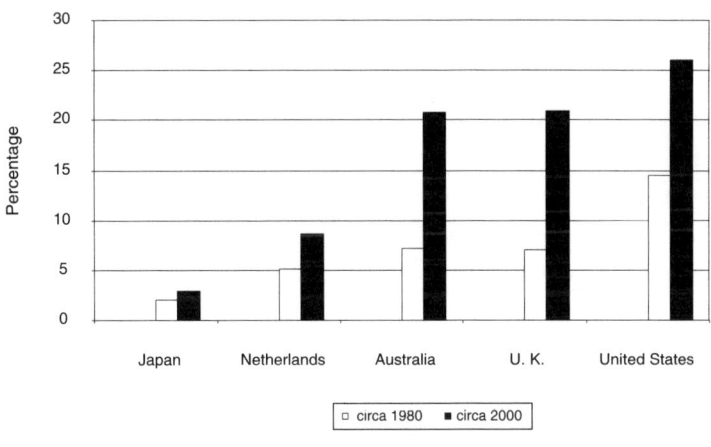

SOURCE: OECD 2003.

deaths in the United States, ranking number two in lifestyle or consumer choice variables (behind smoking, but well ahead of alcohol consumption).[4]

In a large-scale, multivariate analysis, Roland Sturm (2002) found obesity to have a major impact on health status and health-care use in the United States. Obesity led to far worse performance on two measures of health status. The first was the number of chronic conditions reported (out of a possible total of seventeen), and the second was a physical health scale. In both cases, obesity led to far worse outcomes than smoking, problem drinking, or being merely overweight. In fact, obesity had the same effects on health as an extra twenty or thirty years of aging.

If that finding is not striking enough, consider the effects of obesity on health-care use. Sturm found that obesity led to 36 percent more total health-care consumption and a whopping 77 percent more pharmaceutical consumption. By comparison, smoking, the next most important lifestyle variable, raised total health-care consumption by 21 percent, and pharmaceutical use by 28 percent. Sturm found being overweight to be far less serious than obesity, with statistically insignificant point estimates of less than one-third of the effects of obesity.

Given the growing impact of obesity on health in wealthy nations, some economists have turned their attention to trying to explain why it is on the rise. Tomas Philipson and Richard Posner (1999) have argued that technical change has encouraged the increase in obesity by making it easier and cheaper to consume calories, while at the same time discouraging physical activity by substituting light for heavy work. They analyzed consumers' choice of body weight, explaining the increase in obesity in recent years in a static, fully utility-maximizing framework. This provided a nice example of how powerful standard economic theory is for explaining behavioral changes in response to change in the constraints. Sam Peltzman (2001) recently wrote about health-related behavior that offsets improvement in the productivity of health care, although he did not apply this idea to obesity. He argued that when health risks are reduced, consumers partly cancel out the health gains by pursuing less healthy behavior. Although he pointed to accidents, suicides, and homicides, his ideas may very well apply to obesity. For instance, since most of the important recent improvements in health care have come in fighting circulatory disease, it is possible that consumers have become more likely to choose a sedentary lifestyle and to overeat because they believe modern medicine can bail them out of their resulting health problems.

Obesity, however, is a complex condition. Consumers themselves often voice discontent with their own obesity, possibly making it a problem in the economics of self-control. Consumers' tastes may change over time in inconsistent ways, such that their planned diets may not be carried out.[5]

Trent Smith (2001) has given a very interesting evolutionary interpretation of overeating. He has suggested that the biological mechanisms underlying the sensations of hunger and satiation evolved to serve humans well when they were faced with periodic famines. Now that famines are exceedingly rare in rich countries, the very same biological mechanisms lead to obesity. Consumers are still behaving rationally, overeating when they feel hungry as a way to store calories in preparation for a famine. It is simply that this evolutionary programming leads to excessive fat in today's wealthy countries, where food is plentiful all the time.

Other Studies of the Productivity of Pharmaceuticals

Frank Lichtenberg (2000b, 2001, 2003) has studied the productivity of pharmaceutical innovation in novel ways, exploring variation across diseases within the United States. In one of his studies (2000b), he examined the effect on mortality of using new rather than older drugs. Using data from a large-scale, detailed survey of U.S. consumers that contained three waves of interviews over a short time period to examine the effects of different prescriptions on mortality, he found significantly lower mortality (by the end of the third wave of the study) among the users of new drugs, even when controlling for individual characteristics, including details of the diagnosis. He also found the use of new drugs was related to lower disability and lower spending on other types of health care. It is hard to know how these results translate to the life expectancy or mortality of entire populations, making it difficult to compare this study to ours.

Lichtenberg found similar beneficial effects of newer drugs when he introduced dummy variables for each individual and studied the effect of new drugs on all the measures except mortality. This was even harder to interpret.

Further, omitted variable bias is a major problem in interpreting Lichtenberg's results. Suppose that healthier people, within each diagnosis, were more likely to get the newer drug. This could have happened if the people with milder forms of the illness had only recently been put on drug therapy. Having no history of using the older drug, they might naturally have been given the newer one. In this situation, all of Lichtenberg's results might have been obtained purely because of the correlation between the newness of the drug and the mildness of the illness. On the other hand, people with worse forms of the illness might have received the newer drugs if they were more powerful and more costly. Lichtenberg acknowledged this problem in the paper, but argued that the literature on small area variations (which shows that the amount of health care that people receive for the same diagnosis varies greatly by geographic area) suggested it might be acceptable to treat the data as if they were generated by a random assignment of people to new versus old drugs. This struck us as a big leap.

We found Lichtenberg's 2003 study both easier to interpret and more convincing, though it still could not be directly compared to our work. In this analysis, Lichtenberg related the change in the PYLL from 1970 to 1991 to the proportion of drugs classified as new (FDA approval after 1970) that were prescribed for each diagnosis. Each of the eighty observations was an aggregate diagnosis (ICD9 two-digit level disease). He found strong effects, explaining almost half of the variation. Quantitatively, the effects were large. For the quartile with the highest new drug use, the PYLL declined by 72.7 percent. For the quartile with the lowest new drug use, the PYLL declined by only 13 percent.

These results indicated that drug research is highly productive of better health. Using a conservative value of $25,000 per life year saved and an average cost of $667 million for a new drug approval, Lichtenberg found the social rate of return from pharmaceutical innovation to be about 40 percent.[6] While not directly comparable to our results on the consumption of pharmaceuticals, this was certainly consistent with our finding that more consumption raises life expectancy. Also note that in the calculation of the social rate of return from pharmaceutical innovation, Lichtenberg ignored the fact that the innovations benefited consumers in the entire world, not merely the United States. As in the choice of a dollar value per life year, this was a conservative approach. Adjusting for the worldwide health benefits would have attributed even higher benefits to pharmaceutical research and development.

3

Extending Our Earlier Work on Pharmaceutical Consumption

As we have already stated, our prior research showed that people living in countries with higher per-capita pharmaceutical consumption could expect to live longer lives than those in countries with lower consumption rates. These results left us with more questions to consider.

- Does pharmaceutical or other health-care consumption have a bigger effect on the quality of life than on the length of life?
- What effects do they have on the likelihood that an individual will die of any particular common disease?

To answer these questions, we first replicated our original research, with newer data and a slightly improved model that allowed us to take account of the large international variation in obesity. Then we applied our models to disability-adjusted life expectancy as a way to measure the effects of health care on quality of life. Finally, we analyzed how the effects of health care varied by cause of death.

To analyze the impact of health care on life expectancy, we added several measures of health that were not included in our original research: quality of life (as measured by disability-adjusted life expectancy); premature mortality due to circulatory disease, cancer, and respiratory disease (as measured by potential years of life lost); and, finally, mortality rates by age group due to those classes of disease. The following sections explain how these measures were calculated, and our reasons for choosing them.

Quality of Life

Simple measures of life expectancy, used in our earlier study as one means of measuring health, have the benefits of being objective and easy to compare across countries. However, people consume pharmaceuticals not just to live longer lives, but to enjoy better health—a better quality of life. The process of finding appropriate measures of quality of life with respect to health is full of pitfalls, but it is essential to studying the effects of pharmaceutical consumption.

Mortality-based measures such as life expectancy miss completely the morbidity dimension of health that is, we believe, more sensitive to pharmaceutical consumption and other health care.[7] Of course, there are a number of direct morbidity measures, such as workdays lost or subjective evaluations of health. Many are so partial and context-specific that they can't even be meaningfully compared across countries, let alone used in aggregate production of health analysis.

Therefore, we believe the best way to study the relationship between pharmaceutical consumption and quality of life is to use yet another class of health measures. The basic idea behind these measures is to adjust life span either for premature death or the amount of time spent in imperfect health. When the focus is on years lost or gained, the measure is called quality-adjusted life years (QALYs). QALYs are created by multiplying the number of life years by a weight reflecting the quality of life (the opposite of morbidity) (Johannesson 1996, 117–218).

There are many approaches to finding the weights to employ. Ideally, researchers conduct surveys, asking people how they value various aspects of health. They then adjust life expectancy by a certain amount based upon the survey responses. Other QALY measures use weights derived from the opinions of researchers, such as physicians, or from other types of surveys in which individuals are not asked to choose among specific health states. All the methods are problematical, not least because estimating the weights requires sophisticated multidimensional measurement and weighing of quality of life (Bowie et al. 1997). The measures are particularly difficult to interpret across cultures and across long periods of time. At best, QALYs can approximate the number of healthy years people can expect to live.

Another measure is called disability-adjusted life years (DALYs). This measure starts with a baseline of a person living some number of years, assumed to be a full life span, with no disabilities. Then researchers adjust that age for the specific amount of time assigned to each given disability. This measure focuses on disability as a way of reducing the dimensionality of the quality measures.

When applied to life expectancy, this approach yields the disability-adjusted life expectancy (DALE). The WHO, as part of its global burden of disease project, has used this approach to calculate DALEs for most of the countries in the world. These measures are designed for aggregate comparisons of the burden of disease and studies of resource allocation in health care. Both the method of construction and the purpose of the measures are described and defended by Christopher Murray and Arnab Acharya (1997).

A reasonable measure available across countries, the DALE is constructed by a group of health-care providers (mostly physicians) who meet in Geneva to assign weights to each different disability. The weights thus reflect the altruistic or social values of this group, rather than the preferences of the consumers themselves.[8] Weights differ by age, with higher weights for young adults (Murray and Acharya 1997, 712–19). Further, future ill health is discounted at 3 percent. An alternative measure of DALYs uses zero percent discounting and equal age weights. However, when the two measures are applied to calculate the burden of diseases, they are highly correlated across diseases (Murray and Acharya 1997, 719–26), meaning that, for the purposes of this study, the use of the former measure should pose no controversy.

Cause-Specific Mortality

Yet another measure is mortality due to different causes. The WHO regularly collects mortality data from over one hundred countries. Mortality rates are available by cause and are disaggregated by age and gender. For instance, the data set contains information on lung cancer mortality among French men ages sixty-five to seventy-four, and on ischemic heart disease mortality for Swedish women ages fifty-five to sixty-four.

The PYLL measure, which was mentioned earlier, is calculated from the WHO's age- and gender-specific mortality rates. PYLL represents the difference between a fixed measure of potential life span (which varies by study, mostly between sixty-five and eighty-five years) and the time of actual death, making it in effect a weighted mortality rate. Note that the extension of life after the fixed potential life span is implicitly given a value of zero using this measure.

If one had data on a panel of countries over time, PYLL would be expressed algebraically as a rate per 100,000 population as

$$(1) \quad PYLL = \sum_{a=0}^{l-1} (l - a)(d_{at}/p_{at})(P_a/P_n)*100{,}000,$$

where:

a = age,
l = the age limit,
d_{at} = the number of deaths at age a,
p_{at} = the number of persons aged a in country i at time t,
P_a = the number of persons aged a in the country,
P_n = the total number of persons aged 0 to l-1 in the country.

This measure is very useful because, unlike data on life expectancy, it is well defined for different causes of death. Using WHO mortality data, the OECD routinely calculates PYLL measures for a number of different causes of death, setting seventy years as its age limit.

In this study, we focused on the most prevalent causes of death in twenty of the twenty-one OECD countries that we had included in our previous analysis. (Data limitations forced us to leave Turkey out of our present analyses.[9]) Table 1 shows the average mortality rates (per 100,000 population) among the twenty countries for fourteen different causes of death. We found, not surprisingly, that circulatory disease was the leading cause of death in these countries, accounting for 40 percent of all deaths in 1994. Cancer was the second leading cause of death, accounting for 26 percent, and respiratory disease was a distant third, accounting for 8 percent. Taken together, these three causes accounted for about three-quarters of all deaths in 1994. Because of their prevalence, we used these cause-specific mortalities in our present study.

Table 1: Leading Causes of Death in Twenty OECD Countries, 1994

Cause of Death	Mortality Rate[a] OECD Mean	Percentage of Total Mortality
All causes	739.3	100.0
Circulatory diseases	294.7	39.9
Cancers	195.1	26.4
Respiratory diseases	59.8	8.1
Digestive system diseases	30.6	4.1
Endocrine and metabolic disorders	29.8	4.0
Nervous system diseases	14.2	1.9
Mental conditions	11.8	1.6
Genito-urinary conditions	10.8	1.5
Infectious diseases	8.0	1.1
Congenital anomalies	4.4	0.6
Musculoskeletal conditions	3.0	0.4
Diseases of the blood	2.6	0.4
Diseases of the skin	1.1	0.1
Other causes	73.5	9.9

SOURCE: Authors' calculations using OECD (2000) data.
a. Measured as number of deaths per 100,000 in the population.

4

Modeling the Production of Health

The following sections describe our model and the data we used as inputs. Our model started with the assumption that people consume health-care goods and services and choose certain environmental and lifestyle factors. Together, these factors combine to produce a certain level of health five to ten years later than when they were consumed. The idea here is that many factors, such as smoking, will not have a measurable impact on an individual's health until some time in the future. We then applied this assumption to national populations to analyze how health levels differed from country to country.

In this section, we provide specifics on the model and data we used in this study. We also discuss how we measured health care, with further discussion of the crucial issue of the specific purchasing power parity rates that we used to convert drug prices to common terms.

Our Model

As in our previous work, we based our analysis on the standard household production model of health, in which the level of an individual's health is determined by his or her consumption of medical-care goods and services as well as wealth and environmental and lifestyle factors. Aggregating up to the national level yielded the following model to explain the variation in health levels across countries:

$$(2)\ H_i = \alpha + \beta MC_i + \varphi\, W_i + \gamma X_i + \varepsilon_i,$$

where H_i is the measure of the average health of the citizens of country i,

24

MC_i is a vector of the average consumption of various types of medical care by the citizens of country i, W_i is per-capita wealth of country i, X_i is a vector of lifestyle or environmental variables for country i, and ε_i is a random error term.

Data Sources

The data we used in this study came from two sources. Most were from the 2000 release of the OECD's Health Data database (see OECD 2000). The OECD collects data from member countries, including broad health system outcomes measures, such as life expectancies and infant mortality, as well as total and public expenditures on various health-care inputs, including pharmaceuticals. To facilitate cross-national comparisons, various exchange rates are provided to convert these health-care expenditure levels into U.S. dollars. The OECD provides separate PPP exchange rates for both total medical services and pharmaceuticals for the years 1980, 1985, 1990, 1993, and 1996. These data are available for almost all countries in the 1990s and for most countries in 1980 and 1985.

The OECD data also include information on various macroeconomic indicators such as GDP, education, and employment. Finally, they include measures of environmental factors expected to affect health, such as alcohol and tobacco consumption, pollutant emissions, and dietary make-up.

Although the OECD generates PYLLs by cause of death, it does not collect disease-specific mortality data broken out by age and gender, so we instead used data compiled by the WHO, which are available on the WHO website (WHO 2003) and in various publications. The DALE data produced as part of the WHO's global burden of disease project were also provided in the WHO's World Health Report 2000 (see Murray and Acharya 1997).

Health Indicators

As stated in the last section, we used a new set of health indicators in this study. We estimated models for DALE at birth and at age sixty. The DALEs came from the 1998–1999 time period. We also estimated models for life expectancy at birth and at ages forty and sixty, using life expectancy data from 1997 to 1999. We did this for two reasons. First, we wanted to be able to compare the impacts of medical-care inputs and other factors on the life expectancy and DALE measures. Second, the data in this work were newer than in our previous study. Also, we used a slightly different model, so that these results were a check on the robustness of our previous results.

Other new measures included mortality due to circulatory disease, cancer, and respiratory disease. We estimated PYLL models for each of these three leading causes of death, using PYLLs obtained from the OECD. As we mentioned earlier, in calculating PYLLs the OECD considers deaths before the age of seventy to be "preventable," and therefore sets seventy as the potential life span.[10] This is a fairly short life span, so the effects of pharmaceuticals and other health care focused on older consumers would be missed. Because of this limitation, we also examined separate models for cause-specific mortality rates at particular ages: thirty-five to fifty-four, fifty-five to sixty-four, sixty-five to seventy-four, and seventy-five and up. All of these cause-specific mortality measures came from the 1994 to 1996 time period, and the rates were obtained from the WHO. Not surprisingly, the results of the models for the PYLLs were very similar to those for mortality rates at ages thirty-five to fifty-four and fifty-five to sixty-four. Therefore, for the sake of brevity, we do not report results from the models for age-specific mortality rates at ages younger than sixty-five. Instead, we report only the results for the PYLLs, which capture the effects on mortality for the nonelderly, along with the results on the mortalities at ages sixty-five to seventy-four and seventy-five and over, which capture the effects on mortality among the elderly. Note that the effects of inputs that improve health on the age-specific mortality for people of older ages were biased downward. The population base for these age groups includes people who were healthy enough to have survived to these later ages. To see how this could lead to a downward bias on the effect of health care on the elderly, consider this very simple example:

- Scenario One: Suppose the entire population of seventy-year-olds in a country consists of two people. One of these people, due to the luck of the genetic draw, is and has always been very healthy. The other has been less lucky, and has always had health problems. Still, this second person has survived to the age of seventy because she has been able to obtain high-quality health care. Now suppose that in the next year, this less-healthy person dies. This would lead to a mortality rate among seventy-year-olds of 50 percent (one out of the two people in the population died).

- Scenario Two: Now suppose that the entire population of seventy-year-olds in a country consists of one person. This person, due to the luck of the genetic draw, is and has always been very healthy. The second person from Scenario One has not survived to the age of seventy because under this scenario, high-quality health care has not been made available. Since the one person who has survived to the age of seventy is in good health, he does not die over the course of the next year. Under this scenario, the mortality rate among seventy-year-olds is zero. Thus, here is a case where less health care can lead to lower mortality among the elderly. Because the less-healthy individual did not get the necessary care in the past, she never survived to the age of seventy.

Medical-Care Inputs

All explanatory variables are listed in table 2. As in our previous study, we focused here on two medical-care inputs: consumption of pharmaceuticals and consumption of other medical care. The data on consumption came from the OECD (2000).

Based on the results of our previous work, we created a measure of pharmaceutical consumption by converting 1990 per-capita expenditures on pharmaceuticals to U.S. dollars, using pharmaceutical PPP exchange rates also provided by the OECD.[11] We created a measure of other medical-care consumption in two steps. First, we converted 1990 per-capita expenditures on medical care to U.S. dollars using medical-care PPP exchange rates. We then subtracted our pharmaceutical consumption measure from this figure.

In the next section we provide a justification for the validity of these measures. Those readers familiar with our 1999 study can skip this section and move on to our discussion of other explanatory variables.

Table 2: Definitions of Explanatory Variables

FEMALE	An indicator variable equal to 1 if the observation is for a female outcomes measure.
GDPPC	Gross domestic product per capita in 1990, converted to U.S. dollars using the GDP purchasing power parity exchange rate.
PHPC	Pharmaceutical expenditures per capita in 1990, converted to U.S. dollars using the purchasing power parity exchange rate for pharmaceuticals.
HEPC	Other health expenditures per capita in 1990, converted to U.S. dollars using the purchasing power parity exchange rate for health care.
SMOKE	If female = 1, the percentage of females ages 15 and over who smoke; If female = 0, the percentage of males ages 15 and over who smoke.
ALCOHOL	Alcohol consumption circa 1990, measured as liters consumed per capita.
ALCOHOL *FEMALE	ALCOHOL interacted with FEMALE.
OBESITY	If female = 1, the percentage of females with BMI ≥ 30; If female = 0, the percentage of males with BMI ≥ 30.

Measuring Pharmaceutical Consumption

As we have already discussed, how one converts a nation's per-capita pharmaceutical expenditures to U.S. dollars for the purpose of cross-national comparisons is of crucial importance. One could use PPP exchange rates designed to convert total GDP to U.S. dollars. This approach is only appropriate if pharmaceutical prices differ across countries in the same way that prices differ in general. Researchers who have looked at this issue in depth, including Tadeusz Szuba (1986) and Patricia Danzon and Allison Percy (1995), have demonstrated that this is far from the case. Drug price regulation remains a national prerogative in many countries, and trade barriers have traditionally been significant. Both price regulation and barriers vary widely. For instance, France and Italy regulate prices in order to encourage use of pharmaceuticals produced by domestic companies. Other OECD countries, such as the United Kingdom and Germany, also regulate pharmaceutical prices, albeit indirectly and typically much less stringently. The United States and Denmark, at the other extreme, generally permit free pricing of pharmaceuticals, subject to market forces. For these reasons one might expect GDP PPP exchange rates to be unsatisfactory for converting pharmaceutical expenditures to U.S. dollars for cross-national comparisons.

Luckily, PPP exchange rates designed specifically for converting pharmaceutical expenditures to U.S. dollars are available for 1980, 1985, 1990, 1993, and 1996 in the OECD database. In our earlier study, we compared measures of per-capita pharmaceutical expenditures converted to U.S. dollars using pharmaceutical PPP exchange rates and GDP PPP exchange rates. We noted that conversions using the GDP PPP exchange rates invariably underestimated actual pharmaceutical expenditures outside of the United States.

Danzon and Percy (1995) have argued that even the pharmaceutical PPP exchange rates provided by OECD were flawed, and they provided more accurate price indexes for a handful of countries to convert pharmaceutical expenditures to U.S. dollars. These relative price measures should be regarded as the "gold standard," but they are only available for France, Italy, Germany, and the United Kingdom. Szuba (1986) also painstakingly assembled price ratios using detailed proprietary data, though with a slightly different approach. His price coefficients are also excellent, when available.

We compared measures of real pharmaceutical expenditures for 1985 using the following conversion factors: market exchange rates, GDP PPPs, pharmaceutical PPPs, Danzon and Percy's Fisher price indexes, and Szuba's price coefficients. Again we found differences, but a general pattern emerged. France seemed to outspend the other countries significantly. Italy and Germany were at the next tier, with expenditures significantly higher than in the United States. Switzerland and the United Kingdom tended to consume fewer pharmaceuticals than the United States, no matter which measure was used.

We also calculated correlations among the different measures for 1985. The measure generated using OECD's pharmaceutical PPP exchange rate was very highly correlated with both the Danzon and Percy measure and the Szuba measure for the countries for which all of the measures were available. Note that the measures that used simple market exchange rates and GDP PPP exchange rates were not highly correlated with the Danzon and Percy or Szuba measures. These analyses, along with conversations with officers at the OECD, led us to believe that using the pharmaceutical PPP exchange rates would be a significant step forward from other work, which used the GDP PPP exchange rates. Since we wished to study more than the five countries for which Danzon and Percy provided price indexes, the pharmaceutical PPP exchange rates provided by OECD, however imperfect, were the best conversion factors available.

Therefore, our measure of pharmaceutical consumption was the 1990 per-capita pharmaceutical expenditure for each country, converted to U.S. dollars using the PPP exchange rates provided in the OECD database. Similarly, we constructed a measure of health-care consumption in 1990 using health-care-specific PPP exchange rates as described above.

Other Explanatory Variables

We also included four measures of living standards and lifestyle factors in our study:

- We included each nation's 1990 per-capita GDP, converted to 1990 U.S. dollars using each nation's 1990 GDP PPP exchange rate.
- We controlled for cigarette smoking by including the percentages of females and males ages fifteen years or over who smoked as of the period around 1990. As we noted in our previous work, we preferred measuring smoking in this way because most health researchers believe the adverse effects of smoking begin at low levels of consumption. The effect of switching from ten cigarettes a day to two packs a day is small, while the effect of switching from not smoking at all to smoking ten cigarettes a day is large. The percentage of the population that smokes captures this inherent nonlinearity better than a measure that simply gauges the average tobacco consumption in grams per person per day.

- We controlled for alcohol consumption, which was measured as per-capita consumption in liters. Data on the percentage of adults who consumed alcohol did not exist for enough of the countries in our sample. (For alcohol, unlike smoking, there is not a clear a priori reason to prefer a percentage measure.)
- We controlled for obesity. Our measure was quite standard and newly available for all countries in our sample except Germany and Greece. As discussed above, it was the percentage of the population that was obese, defined as a BMI of thirty or more. At the time of our earlier study, data on obesity levels were quite sparse, so we controlled for richness of diet by including a measure of animal-fat calories consumed per capita per day in an effort to create a proxy for obesity. For the present study, enough data on obesity levels existed to allow us to use the new measure. The only drawback was that we had to drop Germany and Greece from our sample. Still, the models that included obesity levels generally performed better than those that included the animal-fat calorie measures.

Finally, in addition to the living standards and lifestyle variables, we controlled for differences in female and male mortality rates across countries.

The Model Specification and Estimation

We used regression analysis to determine the effect of each of the explanatory variables on each of the health indicators. We lagged the explanatory variables by roughly five to ten years because we believe that lifestyle factors and medical-care consumption have a cumulative rather than an instantaneous effect on health. A full model would have required several lags of each explanatory variable. Due to data and sample size limitations, this was impossible. The implicit assumption we made here was that cross-national variations in the values of the explanatory variables as of 1990 reflected their historical cross-national variations. We checked this assumption in our sensitivity analyses.

As in our previous work, we used a log-log, or constant elasticity, functional form. There are two advantages to this specification. First, a coefficient from a log-log regression is interpreted as an elasticity: the percentage change in the dependent variable associated with a 1 percent change in the value of an explanatory variable. Second, a model for the production of health should allow for diminishing returns to all of the explanatory variables. In the log-log model, the elasticity is held constant and the absolute value of the marginal effect of each explanatory variable is forced to fall at higher and higher values of the explanatory variable. The data to which one applies such a model determine the rate at which the marginal effect decreases.

Finally, in our regression analyses, we pooled our data across sexes and included an indicator variable, FEMALE, equal to one for observations on female health outcomes and zero for observations on male health outcomes. We did this because, as a rule, the effects of the various explanatory variables did not differ significantly by sex except for alcohol consumption. We included an interaction term between the gender indicator variable and alcohol consumption to capture this. It should be noted that SMOKE (see table 2) was equal to the percentage of females who smoked for those observations where FEMALE equaled one and to the percentage of males who smoked for those observations where FEMALE equaled zero. Likewise, OBESITY was equal to the percentage of females who were obese (BMI was thirty or greater) for those observations where FEMALE equaled one and the percentage of males who were obese for those observations where FEMALE equaled zero.

One would have expected mild heteroskedasticity in these data, meaning that the error terms were not identically distributed. Further, because we had pooled observations on male and female health outcomes, there were two observations for each of the eighteen countries in our sample. It was possible, even likely, that the within-country observations were not independent because of unobserved country effects.

These problems did not create bias or inconsistency in the estimated beta coefficients, but they could have led to problems in the estimated standard errors. We corrected for these problems by estimating the standard errors using a version of the robust heteroskedasticity-consistent covariance estimator, which was introduced by R. J. Huber (1967) and further developed by H. White (1980). W. H. Rogers (1993) has noted that one can use a version of this estimator when relaxing the assumptions of both identically and independently distributed error terms. In our case, we needed only assume that the observations were independent across countries.

5

Results

Descriptive Statistics

As the descriptive statistics in tables 3 and 4 show, there was much variation in the cause-specific mortality rates for both men and women among the eighteen OECD countries we used in our final analyses.[12] Although circulatory disease was the leading cause of death in these countries, cancer was actually a greater cause of premature mortality, especially among women. Cancer was the cause of over 1,100 PYLLs (before the age of seventy) per 100,000 women, whereas circulatory disease was the cause of only about 458 PYLLs per 100,000 women. Although the difference was smaller, cancer was the leading cause of premature mortality among men as well. The respiratory disease mortality rates were the smallest, but they also exhibited the greatest variation as measured by their coefficients of variation. Of course, the male mortality rates were mostly higher than the female mortality rates. Another finding from tables 3 and 4 is that DALEs exhibited slightly greater variation than did the life expectancies.

The descriptive statistics shown in table 5 indicated a good deal of variation in the explanatory variables as well. Pharmaceutical consumption per capita, for example, varied by a factor of over six, from $105.20 in Ireland to $664.60 in France. GDP varied by a factor of over two, from $9,598 in Portugal to $22,266 in the United States. Other health-care consumption varied by a factor of almost four, from $714.30 in Portugal to $2,515.00 in the United States. Lifestyles also varied widely in our sample. Men in Spain were twice as likely to smoke as men in Sweden, and women in Denmark were seven times more likely to smoke than women in Portugal. The French consumed more than three times the alcohol per capita than that consumed by the Norwegians.

Table 3: Descriptive Statistics for Outcomes Measures, Females

Outcomes Measure	Average	Standard Error	Minimum	Maximum
Life expectancy (years)				
at birth	80.22	1.22	77.8	81.9
at 40	41.51	1.17	39.0	43.2
at 60	23.23	1.00	21.4	24.9
Disability-adjusted life expectancy (years)				
at birth	74.06	1.59	71.2	76.9
at 60	19.04	1.34	16.6	21.7
Cancer mortality				
PYLL[a]	1,102.24	170.53	825.0	1,484.1
Age 65–74[b]	611.70	117.06	432.5	872.9
Age >74[b]	1,189.10	130.54	981.5	1,465.3
Circulatory disease mortality				
PYLL[a]	457.87	116.85	273.0	741.5
Age 65–74[b]	638.31	153.91	331.3	939.1
Age >74[b]	4,191.79	684.22	3,139.4	5,971.6
Respiratory disease mortality				
PYLL[a]	119.61	47.05	62.0	210.7
Age 65–74[b]	133.27	76.72	51.9	284.3
Age >74[b]	813.73	367.29	377.6	1,754.5

SOURCE: Authors' calculations using OECD (2000) and WHO (2000, 2003) data.
a. Measured as potential years of life lost per 100,000 in the population.
b. Measured as deaths per 100,000 in the population.

Obesity, once again, was particularly interesting. The United States had the highest obesity rates by far, with 25.1 percent of women being obese, more than double the mean of 10.7 percent and 67 percent higher than the next highest, the United Kingdom. The story was similar for men. In the United States, 19.9 percent of adult men were obese, again more than double the mean of 9.49 percent, and 50 percent higher than the next highest, Canada. Several European countries had far lower obesity rates; those for Swedish men and for Swiss women were only 5.4 and 4.7 percent, respectively. It should be noted that our data were from various years in the early 1990s. As discussed above, recent trends have indicated rapid increases in obesity rates worldwide, with the United Kingdom and Australia, in particular, catching up by 2000.

Table 4: Descriptive Statistics for Outcomes Measures, Males

Outcomes Measure	Average	Standard Error	Minimum	Maximum
Life expectancy (years)				
at birth	73.95	1.23	71.0	75.9
at 40	36.19	0.99	34.6	37.6
at 60	18.90	0.82	17.4	20.0
Disability-adjusted life expectancy (years)				
at birth	68.81	1.45	65.9	71.2
at 60	15.48	1.00	13.9	16.8
Cancer mortality				
PYLL[a]	1,308.50	204.79	946.7	1,764.2
Age 65–74[b]	1,113.23	122.06	854.9	1,306.0
Age >74[b]	2,289.34	247.44	1,896.1	2,857.4
Circulatory disease mortality				
PYLL[a]	1,195.17	260.68	760.0	1,639.7
Age 65–74[b]	1,320.73	291.26	801.3	1,978.2
Age >74[b]	4,859.27	741.08	3,558.8	6,498.1
Respiratory disease mortality				
PYLL[a]	192.87	71.28	112.4	333.5
Age 65–74[b]	287.06	99.44	150.8	532.2
Age >74[b]	1,393.63	454.90	659.4	2,583.4

SOURCE: Authors' calculations using OECD (2000) and WHO (2000, 2003) data.
a. Measured as potential years of life lost per 100,000 in the population.
b. Measured as deaths per 100,000 in the population.

Table 6 presents simple correlations among the explanatory variables. Most were not significantly different from zero, although the results appeared to indicate that countries with higher pharmaceutical consumption had lower tobacco use rates among females and higher rates of alcohol consumption overall. Richer countries tended to spend more on nonpharmaceutical health-care goods and services, but surprisingly, not on pharmaceuticals. Male and female obesity rates were highly correlated, whereas male and female tobacco use rates were not. This indicates that certain bad health habits, such as over-eating and a sedentary lifestyle, may be culturally ingrained, whereas others, such as smoking, are not. It is also interesting to note that the male smoking rate was positively correlated with the overall rate of alcohol consumption.

Table 5: Descriptive Statistics for the Explanatory Variables

Variable	Mean	Standard Error	Minimum	Maximum
GDPPC	$16,291.1	$3,188.7	$9,598 (Portugal)	$22,266 (United States)
PHPC	$238.3	$132.3	$105.2 (Ireland)	$664.6 (France)
HEPC	$1,741.1	$474.4	$714.3 (Portugal)	$2,515.0 (United States)
SMOKE				
Female	25.2%	7.6%	5.8% (Portugal)	42.0% (Denmark)
Male	35.2%	6.8%	25.7% (Sweden)	51.5% (Spain)
ALCOHOL	10.8 liters	2.6 liters	5.0 liters (Norway)	16.6 liters (France)
OBESITY				
Female	10.1%	4.8%	4.7% (Switzerland)	25.1% (United States)
Male	9.5%	3.7%	5.4% (Sweden)	19.9% (United States)

SOURCE: Authors' calculations using OECD (2000) data.

Empirical Results for Disability-Adjusted and Unadjusted Life Expectancy

The Effects of Lifestyle and Wealth. Of all the lifestyle variables we considered, obesity had the largest impact on life expectancy and disability-adjusted life expectancy, as the results presented in table 7 show. Countries with higher levels of obesity could expect their populations to live shorter lives and suffer more ill health along the way. The results indicate that lowering obesity levels by 10 percent, from the OECD averages of 10 percent to about 9 percent, would increase disability-adjusted life expectancy at birth by about 0.2 percent and at age sixty by about 0.5 percent. This would raise

Table 6: Simple Correlations among the Explanatory Variables

	GDPPC	PHPC	HEPC	Female Smoke	Male Smoke	Alcohol	Female Obesity	Male Obesity
GDPPC	1.000							
PHPC	0.0929	1.000						
HEPC	0.9274[b]	0.1746	1.000					
SMOKE								
Female	0.3467	−0.4944[b]	0.3733	1.000				
Male	−0.1304	0.121	−0.0545	0.2064	1.000			
ALCOHOL	−0.1134	0.5125[b]	−0.132	−0.1913	0.4089[a]	1.000		
OBESITY								
Female	0.1082	−0.0864	0.0641	−0.2106	−0.3361	−0.0201	1.000	
Male	0.1031	−0.1293	0.0553	−0.0946	−0.2971	−0.0293	0.9206[b]	1.000

SOURCE: Authors' calculations using OECD (2000) data.
a. Correlation is significantly different from zero at the 0.10 level.
b. Correlation is significantly different from zero at the 0.05 level.

the average DALE at birth by about fifty-two days for women and about forty-eight days for men. The average DALE at age sixty would increase by thirty-four days for women and twenty-seven days for men.

Our results also showed that changes in obesity levels had a greater impact on DALEs than they did on normal life expectancies. The 10 percent decrease in obesity rates would increase female life expectancy at birth by forty-four days and male life expectancy at birth by forty-one days. It would also increase life expectancy at age sixty by fifteen days for women and by twelve days for men. Here we have found the marginal effects of obesity on quality of life to be greater than on life expectancy. However, this did not necessarily have to be the case, because the mean value of DALE was lower than that for unadjusted life expectancy.

Perhaps surprisingly, the other lifestyle variables did little to explain differences in life expectancy or DALE from country to country. In these models, the effects of alcohol and tobacco consumption on DALE were both exceeded by the size of the standard errors. The effects of alcohol and tobacco consumption on life expectancy measured in this study were similar to those we estimated in our previous research, where we also found

Table 7: Life Expectancy Regressions (standard errors in parentheses)

Variable	Life Expectancies			DALEs	
	at birth	at 40	at 60	at birth	at 60
FEMALE	0.0479	0.0867	0.1693[b]	0.0337	0.1943
	(0.0288)	(0.0534)	(0.0688)	(0.0438)	(0.1163)
GDPPC	−0.0058	0.0455	0.1033	−0.0058	0.0322
	(0.0259)	(0.0506)	(0.0705)	(0.0373)	(0.1290)
PHPC	0.0086	0.0302[b]	0.0607[b]	0.0186[b]	0.0896[b]
	(0.0068)	(0.0113)	(0.0163)	(0.0079)	(0.0234)
HEPC	0.0228	−0.0087	−0.0263	0.0250	0.0444
	(0.0210)	(0.0347)	(0.0484)	(0.0292)	(0.0937)
SMOKE	−0.0040	−0.0045	0.0064	−0.0071	0.0078
	(0.0109)	(0.0173)	(0.0233)	(0.0123)	(0.0344)
ALCOHOL	−0.0107	−0.0194	−0.0137	−0.0118	−0.0102
	(0.0120)	(0.0215)	(0.0268)	(0.0175)	(0.0442)
ALCOHOL * FEMALE	0.0139	0.0210	0.0171	0.0161	0.0073
	(0.0135)	(0.0250)	(0.0314)	(0.0197)	(0.0515)
OBESITY	−0.0153[b]	−0.0191[a]	−0.0176	−0.0192[b]	−0.0485[b]
	(0.0055)	(0.0098)	(0.0136)	(0.0065)	(0.0163)
CONSTANT	4.2170[b]	3.1540[b]	1.8549[b]	4.0971[b]	1.7176[b]
	(0.1428)	(0.2729)	(0.3819)	(0.1908)	(0.6407)
R-SQUARED	0.928	0.922	0.938	0.872	0.883

SOURCE: Authors' calculations using OECD (2000) and WHO (2000) data.
a. Coefficient is significant at the 0.10 level.
b. Coefficient is significant at the 0.05 level.

small elasticity estimates that were swamped by the standard errors. Our current results for the effect of wealth (GDP) on life expectancy were similar to those we found in our earlier study, but here none of the point estimates were precise enough for us to make much of them. Interestingly, the point estimates for GDP were smaller in the comparable DALE models.

The Effect of Nonpharmaceutical Medical-Care Consumption. We found in this study that nonpharmaceutical medical-care consumption did not have a statistically significant effect on life expectancies at even the 10 percent level of significance. While the effects were larger here than the ones we found in our earlier research, they were still smaller than the standard error. Likewise, nonpharmaceutical medical-care consumption had no statistically significant effect on DALE.

Our estimates of the effects of nonpharmaceutical medical-care consumption changed a great deal depending upon whether per-capita GDP was included or excluded as a variable. This was not surprising, given that these two measures were highly correlated; countries with higher per-capita GDP spent more on medical care, and vice versa. For instance, when we excluded per-capita GDP, the measured effect of nonpharmaceutical health-care consumption jumped from an elasticity of 0.044 to 0.065 and became statistically significant at the 10 percent level. This made it very difficult to tell whether the results stemmed from greater nonpharmaceutical health-care consumption, or the simple fact that the population being considered was wealthier.

The Effect of Pharmaceutical Consumption. By contrast, pharmaceutical consumption had a significant effect both on life expectancy and DALE. Countries that consumed more pharmaceuticals saw their populations live longer and suffer less ill health than those that consumed less. As in our earlier study, we found that pharmaceutical consumption had no discernible effect on life expectancy at birth, but it did have a positive and statistically significant relationship with life expectancy at the ages of forty and sixty. Increasing per-capita pharmaceutical expenditures by 10 percent would increase life expectancy at age forty by 0.3 percent, and at age sixty by 0.6 percent. This would increase life expectancy at age forty by forty-six days for women and forty days for men. Life expectancy at age sixty would increase by fifty-one days for women and forty-two days for men.

These results were consistent with our earlier work, though slightly stronger. In our earlier work, a 10 percent increase in pharmaceutical consumption led to an increase in life expectancy of about 0.2 percent at age forty and about 0.4 percent at age sixty. The newer results were more precise, meaning they exceeded the standard error by an

Table 8: Marginal Effect of Pharmaceutical Consumption on Life Expectancy Measures, Females (days per additional 1990 U.S. dollar spent)

Country	Life Expectancies			DALEs	
	at birth	at 40	at 60	at birth	at 60
Australia	1.29	2.36	2.67	2.61	3.36
Austria	1.27	2.30	2.57	2.56	3.10
Belgium	0.83	1.52	1.73	1.66	2.11
Canada	1.18	2.17	2.50	2.33	2.87
Denmark	2.16	3.81	4.20	4.30	4.98
Finland	1.32	2.39	2.66	2.62	3.17
France	0.39	0.72	0.83	0.79	1.07
Ireland	2.35	4.17	4.53	4.63	5.16
Italy	0.57	1.04	1.17	1.14	1.45
Netherlands	1.94	3.47	3.88	3.88	4.95
New Zealand	1.39	2.53	2.84	2.70	3.10
Norway	1.49	2.71	3.03	2.98	3.79
Portugal	0.99	1.80	1.98	2.00	2.35
Spain	0.89	1.65	1.87	1.79	2.29
Sweden	1.13	2.07	2.34	2.25	2.84
Switzerland	1.35	2.49	2.85	2.69	3.54
United Kingdom	1.36	2.43	2.70	2.72	3.31
United States	1.04	1.87	2.11	2.05	2.51
Average	1.06	1.92	2.16	2.11	2.61

SOURCE: Authors' calculations.

even greater margin (Frech and Miller 1999, 42). Furthermore, the fact that our current study yielded similar results, even when using different data and a slightly different model, lent further strength to this conclusion.

The results were even more striking for disability-adjusted life expectancy. A 10 percent increase in pharmaceutical consumption would increase the DALE at *birth* by 0.2 percent, by fifty days for women and forty-seven days for men. This same 10 percent increase in drug consumption would increase the DALE at age sixty by nearly 0.9 percent, by sixty-two days for women and fifty-one days for men. Pharmaceutical consumption not only prolonged life; it also improved the quality of that life.

Table 9: Marginal Effect of Pharmaceutical Consumption on Life Expectancy Measures, Males (days per additional 1990 U.S. dollar spent)

Country	Life Expectancies			DALEs	
	at birth	at 40	at 60	at birth	at 60
Australia	1.20	2.09	2.20	2.45	2.80
Austria	1.17	1.99	2.10	2.37	2.52
Belgium	0.76	1.31	1.38	1.53	1.70
Canada	1.10	1.92	2.04	2.20	2.43
Denmark	2.02	3.38	3.46	4.04	4.12
Finland	1.20	2.01	2.10	2.39	2.49
France	0.35	0.60	0.66	0.71	0.83
Ireland	2.18	3.67	3.67	4.36	4.32
Italy	0.52	0.91	0.95	1.06	1.18
Netherlands	1.80	3.02	3.08	3.63	3.87
New Zealand	1.30	2.26	2.36	2.54	2.63
Norway	1.38	2.37	2.46	2.74	2.90
Portugal	0.90	1.55	1.62	1.81	1.86
Spain	0.81	1.42	1.53	1.65	1.91
Sweden	1.05	1.84	1.94	2.14	2.43
Switzerland	1.24	2.18	2.33	2.48	2.75
United Kingdom	1.27	2.16	2.22	2.58	2.79
United States	0.95	1.64	1.76	1.91	2.04
Average	0.97	1.67	1.76	1.96	2.12

SOURCE: Authors' calculations.

In tables 8 and 9, we present the marginal effects of pharmaceutical consumption on life expectancies and DALEs for each country. In other words, these data revealed how many extra days a person in each country could expect to live for each additional 1990 U.S. dollar spent on pharmaceuticals. We found that countries like France, which consumed the most pharmaceuticals, stood to gain the least from increased drug consumption, whereas countries that consumed fewer drugs stood to gain more. For instance, increasing pharmaceutical consumption by one dollar would increase the DALE at age sixty in Ireland by 5.2 days for women and 4.3 days for men. In France, such an increase would only improve the DALE at age sixty by 1.1 days for women and 0.8 days for men. The results were similar for all five life expectancy measures.

Table 10: Lifetime Cost of Extending Life (or disability-adjusted life) by One Year, Females (in 1990 U.S. dollars)

Country	Life Expectancies			DALEs	
	at birth	at 40	at 60	at birth	at 60
Australia	23,118	12,835	11,562	10,698	8,810
Austria	23,243	13,043	11,916	10,757	9,391
Belgium	35,844	19,923	17,871	16,588	13,973
Canada	25,384	14,029	12,471	11,750	10,174
Denmark	13,290	7,664	7,158	6,151	5,726
Finland	22,446	12,580	11,508	10,389	9,144
France	78,219	42,890	37,769	36,194	28,266
Ireland	12,384	7,070	6,648	5,733	5,487
Italy	52,722	29,205	26,369	24,399	20,321
Netherlands	15,326	8,621	7,883	7,093	5,952
New Zealand	21,112	11,860	10,788	9,775	9,182
Norway	20,030	11,161	10,142	9,271	7,779
Portugal	29,056	16,481	15,335	13,447	12,243
Spain	33,829	18,591	16,621	15,656	12,942
Sweden	26,585	14,710	13,217	12,305	10,365
Switzerland	22,419	12,320	10,950	10,376	8,420
United Kingdom	21,631	12,242	11,269	10,011	8,775
United States	28,259	15,952	14,486	13,080	11,558
Average	28,054	15,684	14,234	12,984	11,180

SOURCE: Authors' calculations.

Further, additional spending on pharmaceuticals had a larger effect at more advanced ages. As an example, on average across all countries, an additional dollar of pharmaceutical consumption increased the DALE for women by about 2.1 days at birth and about 2.6 days at age sixty.

For tables 10 and 11, we estimated how much it would cost over the course of a lifetime to raise a person's life expectancy and DALE by one year. The results told the same story as those reported in tables 8 and 9. The highest expenditures were necessary in France and Italy—where the marginal effects were smallest—and the lowest were necessary in Ireland and Denmark, where the marginal effects were largest. (See figure 2 for selected countries.) The estimates were fairly conservative because they were based on the assumption that pharmaceutical expenditures

Table 11: Lifetime Cost of Extending Life (or disability-adjusted life) by One Year, Males (in 1990 U.S. dollars)

Country	Life Expectancies			DALEs	
	at birth	at 40	at 60	at birth	at 60
Australia	23,140	13,670	13,356	10,707	10,150
Austria	23,269	14,045	13,863	10,769	11,046
Belgium	35,884	21,532	21,205	16,607	16,517
Canada	25,409	14,948	14,443	11,760	11,583
Denmark	13,302	8,164	8,302	6,157	6,670
Finland	22,475	13,752	13,727	10,403	11,080
France	78,321	46,860	44,850	36,245	34,348
Ireland	12,397	7,562	7,807	5,738	6,325
Italy	52,777	31,354	30,821	24,424	23,821
Netherlands	15,341	9,262	9,373	7,100	7,208
New Zealand	21,131	12,571	12,388	9,784	10,479
Norway	20,051	11,946	11,851	9,281	9,571
Portugal	29,094	17,796	17,840	13,467	14,752
Spain	33,869	20,091	19,323	15,674	14,855
Sweden	26,609	15,634	15,184	12,313	11,673
Switzerland	22,443	13,185	12,709	10,388	10,231
United Kingdom	21,651	13,012	13,061	10,019	10,017
United States	28,292	17,099	16,581	13,094	13,571
Average	28,084	16,830	16,597	12,998	13,140

SOURCE: Authors' calculations.

were constant over the entire lifetimes of the individuals. In reality, spending on pharmaceuticals tended to come later in life.

These estimates for life expectancy showed the same pattern as in our earlier work, although the present study showed that a life year could be saved at even lower cost than we had earlier estimated. To give an example, for forty-year-old females in the United States, the earlier work showed that the cost of an additional year of life expectancy was $21,165 (Frech and Miller 1999, 51). In the newer work, the estimate was $15,952. Note that all of our estimates were well below current estimates for the value of a life year, in the neighborhood of $150,000 in the United States, as discussed above.

Next, we turn to a finer level of detail—the determinants of life years lost and age-specific mortality by cause of death.

Figure 2: Lifetime Cost of Disability-Adjusted Life Year, Males, 1990 Dollars

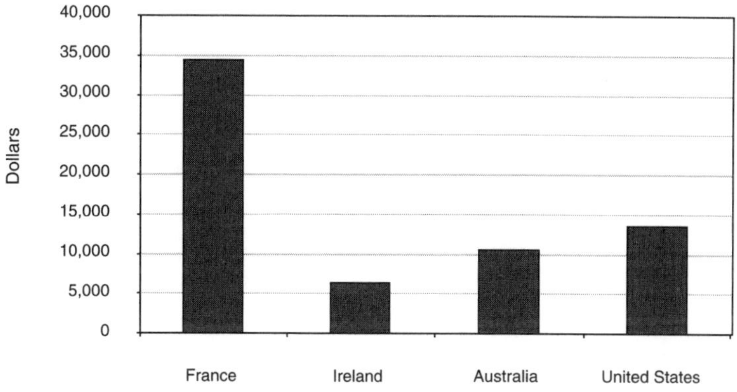

SOURCE: Authors' calculations.

Empirical Results for Circulatory Disease Mortality

The Effects of Lifestyle and Wealth. Table 12 presents our results for circulatory disease mortality, by far the most important cause of death in OECD countries. Not surprisingly, the lifestyle variable with the greatest effect on this type of mortality was obesity. Countries with greater obesity levels also had significantly higher levels of circulatory disease mortality, at least up to the age of seventy-four. Obesity seemed to harm health much more for younger people. Lowering obesity rates by 10 percent, from the sample average of 10 percent to an average of 9 percent, would decrease premature mortality by nearly 4 percent—by nearly eighteen years per 100,000 women and forty-six years per 100,000 men.

Lowering obesity rates by 10 percent would also lower the circulatory disease mortality rate among sixty-five- to seventy-four-year-olds by about 1.6 percent, lowering the average death rates by about ten deaths per 100,000 women and about twenty-one deaths per 100,000 men in this age group. Obesity had little effect on circulatory disease mortality for those ages seventy-five and over. As discussed earlier, the effects on

Table 12: Circulatory Disease Mortality Regressions (standard errors in parentheses)

Variable	PYLL Mean	Mortality Ages 65–74	Mortality Ages > 74
FEMALE	−0.9830[b]	−0.7115[b]	−0.3772
	(0.2961)	(0.2729)	(0.2421)
GDPPC	−0.1628	0.0018	0.3649
	(0.4160)	(0.4177)	(0.2895)
PHPC	−0.1912[b]	−0.3597[b]	−0.1542[b]
	(0.0582)	(0.0680)	(0.0597)
HEPC	0.0134	−0.1034	−0.3479
	(0.2583)	(0.2787)	(0.2109)
SMOKE	−0.0596	−0.1123	−0.1718[b]
	(0.0770)	(0.0928)	(0.0754)
ALCOHOL	−0.1270	−0.1703[a]	−0.0580
	(0.1162)	(0.0925)	(0.1015)
ALCOHOL *FEMALE	−0.0088	−0.0301	0.0707
	(0.1353)	(0.1245)	(0.1126)
OBESITY	0.3861[b]	0.1608[b]	−0.0692
	(0.0822)	(0.0670)	(0.0475)
CONSTANT	9.2313[b]	10.2879[b]	9.2515[b]
	(2.1978)	(2.1271)	(1.4069)
R-SQUARED	0.932	0.907	0.553

SOURCE: Authors' calculations using OECD (2000) and WHO (2003) data.
a. Coefficient is significant at the 0.10 level.
b. Coefficient is significant at the 0.05 level.

mortality of the elderly were biased downward, especially where there was a large effect at the younger ages.

Alcohol consumption may have reduced circulatory disease mortality. This effect held true for men and women ages sixty-five to seventy-four, but the results for people ages seventy-five and over were not statistically significant. Nor did we find a clear effect of alcohol consumption on premature mortality. In our earlier work, alcohol consumption actually led to lower life expectancy (in other words, an increase in overall mortality). We found this surprising, given epidemiological research showing that moderate drinking substantially reduces the risk of heart disease. Now that we are able to reveal the effects of alcohol consumption on different diseases, we can begin to solve this puzzle, as it appears that alcohol consumption does reduce mortality due to heart and circulatory disease.

We could not form clear conclusions about the effects of smoking on circulatory disease mortality, except for those over seventy-four years of age. For this age group, we found smoking reduced circulatory disease mortality. This finding is puzzling and needs to be treated with caution because it is the result of a model with relatively poor fit. (The R-square statistic was only 0.55, whereas the other models boasted R-squares of over 0.90.)

The effects of wealth on circulatory disease mortality were not significant.

The Effect of Nonpharmaceutical Medical-Care Consumption. Nonpharmaceutical medical-care consumption had no statistically significant effect on premature circulatory disease mortality (PYLL), even at the 10 percent level. The effect was fairly large (an elasticity of –0.35) for the oldest age group, and almost significant at the 10 percent level. Still, the results of this model changed substantially when the variable of per-capita GDP was included or excluded. As we have stressed, this showed the need for caution in interpreting the results for either variable. Because countries that had higher per-capita GDPs tended to spend more on nonpharmaceutical health-care consumption, it was hard to tell which variable was producing the observed effects.

The Effect of Pharmaceutical Consumption. Consistent with the widely held view that medical advances have been especially successful in treating circulatory disease,[13] countries in our study with greater pharmaceutical consumption saw less premature mortality due to this class of disease. Likewise, greater pharmaceutical consumption reduced mortality due to circulatory disease among the elderly. Increasing per-capita pharmaceutical consumption by 10 percent, from about $238 to about $262, would decrease the potential years of life lost before seventy by nearly 2 percent—

Figure 3: The Marginal Effect of Pharmaceutical Consumption on Premature Circulatory Disease Mortality, 1990

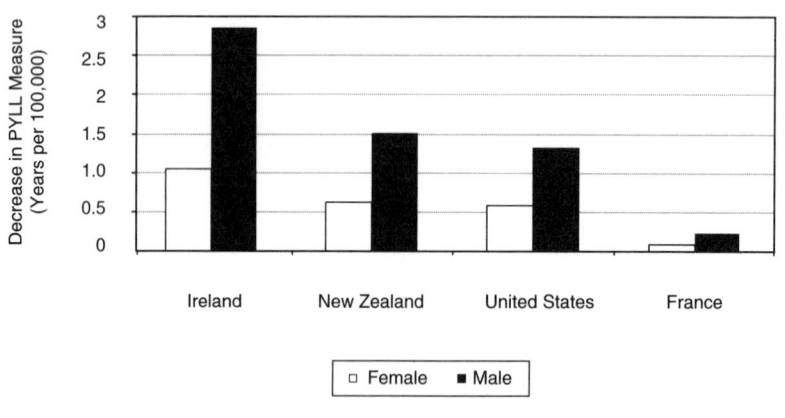

SOURCE: Authors' calculations.

by about nine years per 100,000 women and about twenty-three years per 100,000 men. Such an increase in per-capita pharmaceutical consumption would also lower the circulatory disease mortality rate among sixty-five to seventy-four-year-olds by about 3.6 percent, decreasing the average death rates by about twenty-three deaths per 100,000 women and about forty-seven deaths per 100,000 men in this age group. For those seventy-five and over, the effect was smaller but unambiguous. A 10 percent increase in pharmaceutical consumption would lower mortality rates in this age group by about 1.5 percent, decreasing the average death rates by about sixty-four deaths per 100,000 women and about seventy-five deaths per 100,000 men.

Figures 3 and 4 show the marginal effects of pharmaceutical consumption on circulatory disease mortality in Ireland, New Zealand, the United States, and France. In figure 3, we show the effect on the PYLL measure—in other words, the decrease in premature mortality associated with each additional dollar spent on pharmaceuticals in 1990. Once again, those countries that had already spent the most on pharmaceuticals stood to gain the least by increasing drug consumption, while those that spent the least stood to gain bigger decreases in premature mortality. For instance, in

Figure 4: The Marginal Effect of Pharmaceutical Consumption on Circulatory Disease Mortality among the Elderly, 1990

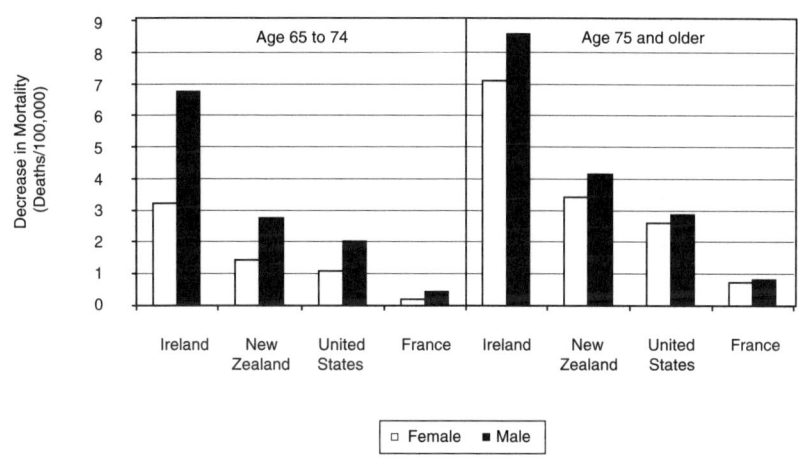

SOURCE: Authors' calculations.

France an additional dollar spent per capita on pharmaceuticals would decrease the PYLL measures by only 0.10 years per 100,000 women and 0.24 years per 100,000 men. In contrast, an additional dollar spent on pharmaceuticals in Ireland would decrease the PYLL measures by about one year per 100,000 women and by nearly three years per 100,000 men.

In figure 4, we focus on circulatory disease mortality rates for those in the sixty-five to seventy-four and seventy-five years and over age groups. It shows the decreases in the mortality rates (per 100,000 individuals) per additional dollar spent on pharmaceuticals in 1990. Generally, the same pattern followed here as in the case of premature mortality, with the higher-drug-consumption countries like France standing to gain less in marginal terms than low-drug-consumption countries. We see here that the marginal effect of drug consumption on circulatory disease mortality was universally higher for men and for those in the seventy-five and over age group. It is also worth noting that pharmaceutical consumption had larger marginal effects on circulatory disease than on overall health.

Table 13: Cancer Mortality Regressions (standard errors in parentheses)

Variable	PYLL	Mortality Ages 65–74	Mortality Ages > 74
FEMALE	0.6594[a]	0.0188	−0.5671[b]
	(0.3355)	(0.2670)	(0.2086)
GDPPC	−0.6205[b]	−0.2832	−0.6373[b]
	(0.1983)	(0.2459)	(0.1922)
PHPC	0.0528	−0.1106[a]	−0.1052[b]
	(0.0548)	(0.0598)	(0.0328)
HEPC	0.2457[b]	0.2246	0.4688[b]
	(0.1211)	(0.1716)	(0.1374)
SMOKE	0.2549[b]	0.2444[b]	0.1060[b]
	(0.1011)	(0.0810)	(0.0487)
ALCOHOL	0.2370[b]	0.1933[b]	0.1443[a]
	(0.1123)	(0.0845)	(0.0730)
ALCOHOL *FEMALE	−0.3153[b]	−0.2307[a]	−0.0213
	(0.1548)	(0.1251)	(0.0913)
OBESITY	0.1568[b]	0.1465[b]	0.0485
	(0.0363)	(0.0330)	(0.0341)
CONSTANT	9.2624[b]	7.0373[b]	10.1653[b]
	(1.1648)	(1.3556)	(0.9838)
R-SQUARED	0.682	0.926	0.964

SOURCE: Authors' calculations using OECD (2000) and WHO (2003) data.
a. Coefficient is significant at the 0.10 level.
b. Coefficient is significant at the 0.05 level.

Empirical Results for Cancer Mortality

The Effects of Lifestyle and Wealth. We present our results for cancer mortality in table 13. In this case, lifestyle variables had a much clearer impact on mortality than they did for circulatory disease.

Given the epidemiological research tying tobacco use to many forms of cancer, it is not surprising to find smoking having a tremendous effect on cancer mortality at all ages. Lowering the smoking rate by 10 percent (from the sample averages of 25.2 percent for females and 35.2 percent for males to 22.7 and 31.7 percent, respectively) would decrease the potential years of life lost before seventy by 2.5 percent. This same decrease in smoking rates would lower cancer mortality by 2.5 percent among those ages sixty-five to seventy-four and about 1 percent among those ages seventy-five and over.

Alcohol consumption was also associated with higher rates of cancer mortality, at least among men. Decreasing alcohol consumption by 10 percent would decrease the potential years of life lost before seventy by about 2.4 percent for men and 1.9 percent among men ages sixty-five to seventy-four. However, alcohol consumption had no effect on either premature mortality or mortality between the ages of sixty-five and seventy-four for women. For both men and women, a 10 percent decline in alcohol consumption would lower the cancer mortality rate among those in the seventy-five and over age group by about 1.4 percent. Again, these results were not terribly surprising, since alcohol consumption is also known to be a contributing factor to certain types of cancer.

More obesity also led to higher cancer mortality rates, at least up to the age of seventy-four. For example, lowering obesity rates by 10 percent, from the sample average of 10 percent to an average of 9 percent, would decrease the potential years of life lost before seventy by about 1.6 percent. This same decrease would also decrease the cancer mortality rate among individuals in the sixty-five to seventy-four age group by roughly 1.5 percent.

Richer countries had lower cancer mortality rates than poorer ones when the other lifestyle factors were held constant. A 10 percent increase in per-capita wealth would decrease the potential years of life lost to cancer before the age of seventy by about 6.2 percent, with a similar effect among those ages seventy-five and over. However, we still faced the same problem with the high correlation between per-capita GDP and nonpharmaceutical consumption, which undermined our confidence in this set of results.

The Effect of Nonpharmaceutical Medical-Care Consumption. Here the results of our models were puzzling. We found greater nonpharmaceutical medical-care consumption related to an increase in cancer mortality, a result that was statistically significant. However, we were skeptical of this result for the same reason explained earlier: the high correlation between per-capita GDP and medical-care consumption. Implausibly large opposite sign coefficients sometimes occur when there is colinearity

Figure 5: The Marginal Effect of Pharmaceutical Consumption on Cancer Mortality among the Elderly

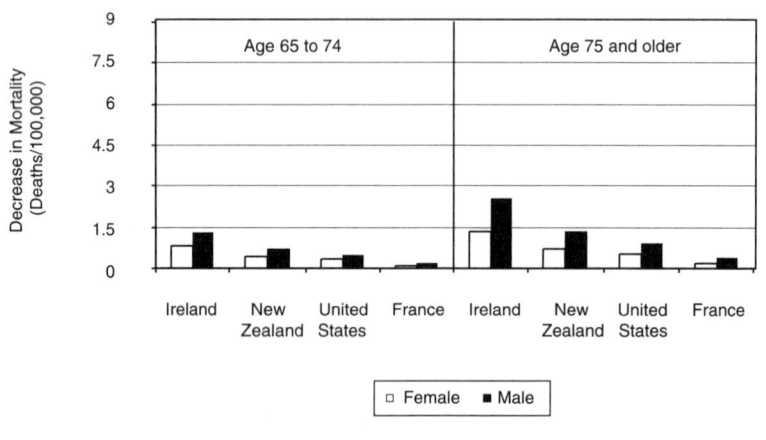

SOURCE: Authors' calculations.

among variables.[14] Indeed, when we excluded the per-capita GDP variable from the model, the result was just the opposite: there was no positive effect of per-capita medical consumption. In our tests of the effects of per-capita GDP on cancer mortality, the results were similarly sensitive to whether the nonpharmaceutical medical-care consumption variable was included or excluded. When we excluded nonpharmaceutical medical-care consumption from the model, what had been a large negative effect of GDP almost vanished. This told us that it was simply impossible to disentangle the effects of per-capita wealth and per-capita nonpharmaceutical medical consumption on cancer mortality.

The Effect of Pharmaceutical Consumption. Pharmaceutical consumption had no statistically significant effect on premature cancer mortality, but it clearly reduced cancer mortality among the elderly. For those seventy-five and over, a 10 percent increase in pharmaceutical consumption would lower the average death rates by about thirteen deaths per 100,000 women and about twenty-four deaths per 100,000 men, a result with strong statistical significance. For those sixty-five to seventy-four, increasing per-capita pharmaceutical consumption by 10 percent would also lower the cancer mortality rate by a little over 1 percent, decreasing the average death rates by about seven deaths per 100,000 women and about twelve deaths per 100,000 men in this age group.

In figure 5 we present marginal effects of pharmaceutical consumption on cancer mortality among the elderly in Ireland, New Zealand, the United States, and France. The same general pattern we saw with circulatory disease emerged. The higher drug consumption countries, such as France, stood to gain less from increasing their spending on pharmaceuticals than low-consumption countries did. For instance, among the sixty-five to seventy-four-year-olds in France, increasing per-capita pharmaceutical consumption by one dollar would lower cancer mortality for males by only 0.37 deaths per 100,000 and for females by only 0.18 deaths per 100,000. In contrast, the corresponding decreases in male and female mortality in Ireland were 1.27 and 0.81 deaths per 100,000. Furthermore, the marginal effect varied by gender and age, being greater for men and for those ages seventy-five and over. Comparing these marginal effects of drug consumption with those we found for circulatory disease in figure 4, we found the marginal effect on circulatory disease mortality generally much higher than the one on cancer mortality.

Empirical Results for Respiratory Disease Mortality

The Effects of Lifestyle and Wealth. Table 14 presents our results for respiratory disease mortality. Not surprisingly, obesity had a very significant effect at all ages. For instance, lowering obesity rates by 10 percent, from the sample average of 10 percent to an average of 9 percent, would decrease premature mortality by about 1.4 percent—by nearly two years per 100,000 women and nearly three years per 100,000 men.

The effect was much bigger for mortality among those ages sixty-five to seventy-four. Lowering obesity rates by 10 percent would also lower the respiratory disease mortality rate in this age group by nearly 7 percent, decreasing the average death rates by about nine deaths per 100,000 women and about twenty deaths per 100,000 men. The effect was also large

Table 14: Respiratory Disease Mortality Regressions (standard errors in parentheses)

Variable	PYLL Mean	Mortality Ages 65–74	Mortality Ages > 74
FEMALE	0.0504	0.3112	−0.1676
	(0.1030)	(0.6537)	(0.6295)
GDPPC	0.1563[a]	−0.5702	−1.5299[a]
	(0.0732)	(0.6142)	(0.6335)
PHPC	0.0075	−0.3352[a]	−0.1531
	(0.0188)	(0.1362)	(0.1277)
HEPC	−0.2041[a]	−0.0693	0.4982
	(0.0480)	(0.4524)	(0.4881)
SMOKE	0.0626[a]	0.6467[a]	0.3224[a]
	(0.0284)	(0.2176)	(0.1619)
ALCOHOL	0.0072	−0.1003	−0.3383
	(0.0332)	(0.2050)	(0.2229)
ALCOHOL *FEMALE	−0.0555	−0.4060	−0.1261
	(0.0484)	(0.3082)	(0.2863)
OBESITY	0.1403[a]	0.6856[a]	0.3723[a]
	(0.0158)	(0.0934)	(0.1013)
CONSTANT	1.0621[a]	9.8795[a]	17.9606[a]
	(0.3985)	(3.1533)	(3.2147)
R-SQUARED	0.836	0.857	0.714

SOURCE: Authors' calculations using OECD (2000) and WHO (2003) data.
a. Coefficient is significant at the 0.05 level.

for those ages seventy-five and over. For this age group, a 10 percent decrease in obesity rates would lower respiratory disease mortality by about 3.7 percent, decreasing the average death rates by about thirty deaths per 100,000 women and about fifty-two deaths per 100,000 men.

Alcohol consumption had virtually no effect on premature respiratory disease mortality, and there was no evidence that this result varied with gender.

Given the epidemiological evidence tying tobacco use to many forms of respiratory disease, especially emphysema, it was not surprising to find smoking raising respiratory disease mortality rates at all ages. A 10 percent decrease in the rate of smoking, from the sample averages of 25.2 percent for females and 35.2 percent for males to 22.7 and 31.7, respectively, would decrease the potential years of life lost before seventy by 0.6 percent. This same 10 percent decrease in smoking rates would have a much bigger effect on respiratory disease mortality among those ages sixty-five to seventy-four, decreasing it by roughly 6.5 percent. It would also decrease the mortality rate among those seventy-five and over by about 3.2 percent.

The findings on wealth were somewhat puzzling. Taken at face value, they suggested that increased wealth had mixed effects on respiratory disease mortality. It was associated with higher premature mortality, but lower mortality among those in the seventy-five and over age group. This suggests that increasing a nation's wealth by 10 percent would lower respiratory disease mortality among the elderly by 15 percent! Again, though, this result was very sensitive to whether we included the variable of nonpharmaceutical medical-care consumption. When this measure was excluded from the model, the effect of per-capita GDP was cut in half.

The Effect of Nonpharmaceutical Medical-Care Consumption. Non-pharmaceutical medical-care consumption lowered premature respiratory disease mortality when we used the PYLL measures. The results indicated that increasing nonpharmaceutical medical care consumption by 10 percent would lower premature mortality by about 2 percent. However, when we studied different age groups, we were left with no statistically significant conclusions as to its effects on anyone over the age of sixty-five. And, again, our results changed significantly when we excluded per-capita GDP. For instance, when we excluded it from the model for mortality at ages seventy-five and over, we found a strong and significant negative effect on mortality. Some combination of wealth and health-care consumption lowered mortality due to respiratory disease for these older individuals, but it was hard to tell which variable produced the effect.

The Effect of Pharmaceutical Consumption. Pharmaceutical consumption had little or no effect on premature respiratory disease mortality, but it reduced respiratory disease mortality among some of the elderly.

Figure 6: The Marginal Effect of Pharmaceutical Consumption on Respiratory Disease Mortality, Ages 65–74

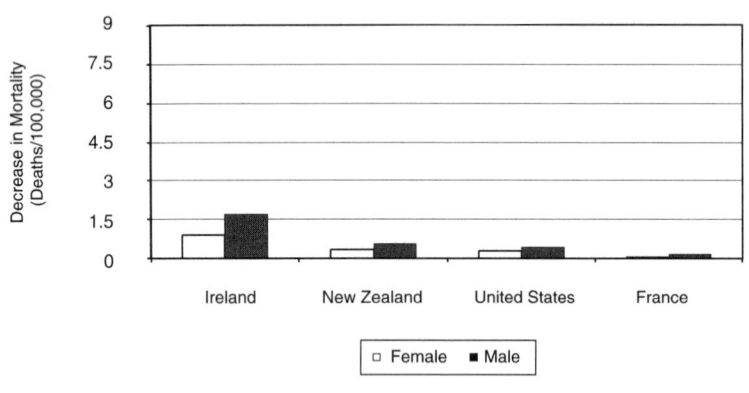

SOURCE: Authors' calculations.

Increasing per-capita pharmaceutical consumption by 10 percent would lower the mortality rate among sixty-five to seventy-four-year-olds by about 3.3 percent, decreasing average death rates by about 4.5 deaths per 100,000 women and about ten deaths per 100,000 men in this age group. The effect was not statistically significant for those seventy-five and over.

In figure 6 we present marginal effects of pharmaceutical consumption on respiratory disease mortality among those ages sixty-five to seventy-four in Ireland, New Zealand, the United States, and France. The same pattern followed here as in the cases of circulatory disease and cancer mortality among these populations, with the higher-drug-consumption countries like France standing to gain less in marginal terms than low-consumption countries. We also saw here that the marginal effect of drug consumption on respiratory disease mortality, as for the other causes of death, was universally higher for men. Comparing across causes of death, we found the marginal effect on circulatory disease mortality generally much higher than the effects on either cancer or respiratory disease mortality.

Sensitivity Testing

We tested our models in many different ways to make sure that our results did not stem from some artifact of the variables we chose or other assumptions we made in building the models. With several exceptions noted below, we found our results to these tests robust, leaving us with even greater confidence in their accuracy.

We have already discussed one possible sensitivity test in previous sections. Our data showed that per-capita GDP and nonpharmaceutical health-care consumption were highly correlated. When we tried to estimate the effects of one measure, the results of our models changed upon including or excluding the other, and caution was needed in interpreting them.

We also varied our models in several ways to see if the results changed. For instance, as we did in our previous study (Frech and Miller 1999), we dropped the lifestyle variables from the models. Just as we found in our earlier research, the effects of pharmaceutical consumption were typically robust to this change. A minor exception was in the respiratory disease model. When we did not control for lifestyle variables, pharmaceutical consumption had a stronger negative effect on respiratory disease mortality.

Our models also assumed we would be able to observe the effects of, say, pharmaceutical consumption on health some eight to ten years later than the date of consumption. To check whether our results were simply the result of an incorrect assumption about the lag time needed to observe these effects, we ran each of the models using explanatory variables from around 1993 and 1996, a lag time of zero to three years. The effects of pharmaceutical consumption did not change in any meaningful way when we made these variations. The observed effects of nonpharmaceutical health-care consumption changed a bit more but were still difficult to interpret due to the colinearity with per-capita GDP.

We also ran our models with additional variables—mean years of education, unemployment, income inequality, and air pollution (as measured by nitrous oxide emissions). Of these, two produced significant changes. Countries with greater levels of education had lower premature circulatory disease mortality, and greater nitrous oxide emissions led to higher respiratory disease mortality among the elderly.

Following the example of Or (2000), we also replaced the nonpharmaceutical health-care consumption measure with a per-capita physician measure. This generally had very little impact on the models. The only case where the measure was significant was in the model for respiratory disease mortality for those ages seventy-five and over, where it had a strong negative impact on mortality. The estimated effects of the other variables, especially pharmaceutical consumption, were not overly sensitive to this change. Interestingly, the effect of the per-capita physician measure became quite strong in many cases when we omitted drug consumption as a variable. This raises the possibility that omitted variable bias may partially explain Or's strong results for the productivity of physicians.

6

Conclusion

We found in this study that pharmaceutical consumption does produce better health. Our analyses here confirmed and strengthened the results of our previous research, which also had concluded that drug use was productive. With the results of this study, however, we can go even farther to say that pharmaceutical consumption not only extends life, but also improves its quality.

This is not to say, however, that all health-care consumption is created equal. While our research revealed that countries that consume more pharmaceuticals enabled their people to enjoy longer and healthier lives, the same could not be said for nonpharmaceutical health-care consumption.

Greater pharmaceutical consumption had strong effects on quality of life, as measured by the number of years people could expect to live without disabling health problems. A 10 percent increase in drug consumption brought about a 0.9 percent increase in the DALE of a person aged sixty. That same increase in drug consumption had a significant but smaller effect on DALE at birth. Just as we found in our previous study, greater drug consumption also led to longer life. The effect we measured here was even larger and of greater statistical significance than the one we uncovered in our previous study, but not as strong as the effect of drug consumption on DALE. A 10 percent increase in pharmaceutical consumption would increase life expectancy at age sixty by 0.6 percent. The similarity between the results of our earlier research and those of this study, which included newer data, underscores our confidence in our findings. When it comes to pharmaceutical spending, our research clearly supports the argument of Cutler and Richardson (1997, 262) that many of the benefits of modern health care pertain to quality of life.

In this research, we also examined the effects of health-care consumption on mortality due to the three most common causes of death in wealthy countries: circulatory disease, cancer, and respiratory disease. Pharmaceutical consumption was clearly productive in reducing death rates due to circulatory disease, at all ages. A 10 percent increase in pharmaceutical consumption cut premature circulatory disease mortality (that is, death before age seventy) by almost 2 percent. Likewise, it reduced death rates among those ages sixty-five to seventy-four by about 3.6 percent, and mortality for those seventy-five and over by 1.5 percent. Considering that circulatory disease was the cause of 40 percent of all deaths in the OECD countries in our study, this is an important finding.

Pharmaceutical consumption had less effect on the mortality of those afflicted with cancer or respiratory disease. Still, it did lower cancer mortality among those ages seventy-five and over and respiratory disease mortality among those ages sixty-five to seventy-four.

As we have just mentioned, we did not find similar clear results when it came to other types of health-care consumption. In some cases, our models did reveal an effect of such consumption on health. But we are unable to say with confidence that this effect was the result of such consumption. When we did observe an effect, it was highly sensitive to the inclusion or exclusion of per-capita GDP in the model. This tells us that any effect we observed could have been either the result of greater non-pharmaceutical health-care consumption or of greater wealth, but it does not tell us which.

We also found obesity detrimental to health, leading to shorter life expectancy, poorer quality of life, and far greater mortality from circulatory disease. This was the only variable other than pharmaceutical consumption that had consistently powerful effects on health. We found that a 10 percent reduction in obesity levels would raise disability-adjusted life expectancy at birth by about 0.2 percent and at age sixty by about 0.5 percent. The same reduction in obesity levels would cut premature mortality due to circulatory disease by nearly 4 percent. Given that obesity is extremely high in the United States and on the rise in several other countries, this is also an important finding.

The health benefits of greater pharmaceutical consumption were also shown to be economically significant. In the United States, spending on pharmaceuticals is middling. Our research indicated that life expectancy for a forty-year-old woman, for example, could be raised by a year at the cost of $15,952. Current estimates place the benefit to society of an extra year of life at about $150,000, making this a very meaningful proposition. In fact, all of our estimates of the cost of raising life expectancy by a year stood well below this level.

Taken together, our results suggest several paths for policymakers to follow. The first is that an agenda supporting the development of newer and better pharmaceuticals is likely to be beneficial to residents even of wealthy countries. It should not be surprising that the strongest effects of pharmaceutical consumption were shown in the reduction of circulatory disease mortality, given the many important new drugs that have been developed to fight this class of disease. In the United States, for example, such an agenda might include streamlining the drug approval process to make it easier for new pharmaceuticals to find their way to market. Such an agenda argues against measures aimed at controlling the prices of pharmaceuticals, as such measures will limit the development of further health-improving drugs by reducing the incentives to develop such new drugs in the first place. Our findings also indicate that crude cost control measures on public health spending may well shortchange the public's health. Health-care consumption clearly matters when it comes to improving health, but the type of consumption matters even more. Pharmaceutical consumption clearly produces better health, and it is a cost-effective way to improve health, when comparing the cost of raising drug consumption against the benefits of extending life expectancy. For the United States, this strengthens the case to include coverage of pharmaceuticals in Medicare, the publicly funded health-insurance program for the elderly. Finally, our results show that obesity is—in the United States, and increasingly around the world—a major threat to health, and that individuals seeking longer and healthier lives would do well to control their weight.

This study overturns a long-held conventional wisdom that health-care consumption does not matter when it comes to improving health in wealthy countries. This belief has, for too long, guided reform efforts and cost cuts down the wrong path. With a new appreciation of how health-care consumption improves health, we can now hope for health policy to do just the same.

Appendix

In tables A-1 through A-5, we list the data that we used in our analyses. Table A-1 lists the life expectancy and DALE measures for each of the countries in our sample. The DALE measures were collected by the World Health Organization (2000) and reflect 1999 levels. The life expectancy measures were compiled by the OECD (2000) and reflect 1995 levels.

Tables A-2 through A-4 present the circulatory disease, cancer, and respiratory disease mortality measures for each of our countries. The PYLL measures were compiled by the OECD, and we obtained the age-specific mortality rates from the WHO website. The PYLL measures all reflect 1994 levels. The age-specific mortality rates generally reflect 1995 levels with the following exceptions: For Austria, Canada, Finland, Portugal, Sweden, and the United Kingdom, the mortality rates reflect 1996 levels. The mortality rate for Belgium is for 1994.

Table A-5 presents the explanatory variable measures for the countries in our sample. The per-capita measures for GDP, pharmaceutical expenditures, and other health expenditures are all from 1990, as is the measure for alcohol consumption. The male and female smoking data reflect 1990 levels with the following exceptions: The smoking data for Australia and Spain are from 1989. The smoking data for Austria are for 1991, and the smoking data for Portugal are a linear extrapolation of 1987 and 1995 levels.

Finally, the obesity data are mostly from the early to middle 1990s. For Australia, Finland, and Sweden, they are from 1990. For Austria, the United Kingdom, and the United States, they are from 1991. For France and Switzerland, they are from 1992. For New Zealand and Spain, they are from 1993. For Canada, Denmark, and Italy, they are from 1994. For Norway and Portugal, they are from 1995. For Belgium and the Netherlands, they are from 1997. For Ireland, they are from 1999.

Table A-1: DALEs and Life Expectancies for the Countries in Our Sample

Country	DALEs (years)		Life Expectancy (years)		
	at birth	at 60	at birth	at 40	at 60
			Females		
Australia	75.5	20.2	80.8	42.1	23.7
Austria	74.4	18.7	80.1	41.2	22.9
Belgium	74.6	19.6	80.2	42.0	23.8
Canada	74.0	18.9	81.3	42.5	24.3
Denmark	71.5	17.2	77.8	39.0	21.4
Finland	73.7	18.5	80.2	41.3	22.9
France	76.9	21.7	81.9	43.2	24.9
Ireland	71.7	16.6	78.6	39.8	21.5
Italy	75.4	19.9	81.0	42.3	23.7
Netherlands	74.4	19.7	80.4	41.0	22.8
New Zealand	71.2	17.0	79.5	41.1	23.0
Norway	74.6	19.7	80.8	41.8	23.3
Portugal	72.7	17.7	78.2	40.3	22.0
Spain	75.7	20.1	81.6	43.0	24.3
Sweden	74.9	19.6	81.3	42.4	23.9
Switzerland	75.5	20.6	81.7	43.0	24.5
United Kingdom	73.7	18.6	79.4	40.5	22.4
United States	72.6	18.4	79.2	40.7	22.9
			Males		
Australia	70.8	16.8	75.0	37.2	19.5
Austria	68.8	15.2	73.5	35.7	18.7
Belgium	68.7	15.8	73.6	36.1	18.9
Canada	70.0	16.0	75.3	37.5	19.9
Denmark	67.2	14.2	72.6	34.6	17.6
Finland	67.2	14.5	72.8	34.8	18.1
France	69.3	16.8	73.9	36.3	19.7
Ireland	67.5	13.9	73.0	35.0	17.4
Italy	70.0	16.2	74.6	36.8	19.2
Netherlands	69.6	15.4	74.6	35.7	18.1
New Zealand	67.1	14.4	74.2	36.7	19.1
Norway	68.8	15.1	74.8	36.6	18.9
Portugal	65.9	14.0	71.0	34.8	18.0
Spain	69.8	16.8	74.4	36.9	19.8
Sweden	71.2	16.8	75.9	37.6	19.8
Switzerland	69.5	16.0	75.3	37.6	20.0
United Kingdom	69.7	15.7	74.1	36.0	18.4
United States	67.5	15.0	72.5	35.6	19.1

SOURCES: DALEs from WHO (2000); life expectancies from OECD (2000).

Table A-2: Circulatory Disease Mortality Measures for the Countries in Our Sample

Country	PYLL	Mortality Ages 65–74	Mortality Age 75+
		Females	
Australia	383.7	562.0	3,981.8
Austria	527.1	789.1	5,971.6
Belgium	431.9	606.4	4,067.2
Canada	409.5	515.9	3,272.5
Denmark	470.4	757.2	4,457.5
Finland	467.5	705.1	4,411.8
France	281.7	331.3	3,139.4
Ireland	578.8	939.1	4,832.2
Italy	421.8	542.6	4,445.0
Netherlands	448.6	602.4	3,467.4
New Zealand	583.2	711.6	3,985.4
Norway	399.5	663.7	3,952.3
Portugal	525.6	750.0	5,348.1
Spain	367.3	453.3	3,849.5
Sweden	353.8	578.1	4,250.1
Switzerland	273.0	427.3	3,994.8
United Kingdom	576.8	826.7	4,001.3
United States	741.5	727.7	4,024.4
		Males	
Australia	998.9	1,138.5	4,417.9
Austria	1,393.4	1,529.6	6,498.1
Belgium	1,028.6	1,156.1	4,568.4
Canada	1,044.3	1,096.2	3,950.3
Denmark	1,166.2	1,544.9	5,371.5
Finland	1,635.2	1,700.1	5,192.8
France	828.8	801.3	3,558.8
Ireland	1,567.8	1,978.2	5,837.9
Italy	1,036.9	1,091.0	4,860.5
Netherlands	1,116.1	1,309.7	4,396.0
New Zealand	1,409.7	1,377.2	4,819.6
Norway	1,136.7	1,483.8	5,174.4
Portugal	1,201.9	1,324.5	5,745.4
Spain	1,068.4	914.7	3,873.9
Sweden	1,051.2	1,326.6	5,333.4
Switzerland	760.0	1,059.3	4,612.1
United Kingdom	1,429.2	1,594.5	4,797.8
United States	1,639.7	1,347.0	4,458.0

SOURCES: PYLL from OECD (2000); mortality rates from WHO (2003).

NOTE: PYLL is measured as potential years of life lost per 100,000 in the relevant population. Mortality is measured as number of deaths per 100,000 in the relevant population.

Table A-3: Cancer Mortality Measures for the Countries in Our Sample

Country	PYLL	Mortality Ages 65–74	Mortality Age 75+
		Females	
Australia	1,057.2	597.6	1,130.7
Austria	1,093.1	590.2	1,272.0
Belgium	1,117.7	585.3	1,325.4
Canada	1,138.5	672.3	1,226.4
Denmark	1,484.1	872.9	1,465.3
Finland	836.9	515.3	1,045.3
France	937.9	477.2	1,124.8
Ireland	1,269.3	771.2	1,357.3
Italy	1,039.3	530.3	1,161.5
Netherlands	1,192.1	628.2	1,285.2
New Zealand	1,352.3	719.2	1,222.8
Norway	1,139.6	595.5	1,163.0
Portugal	1,054.4	458.4	990.4
Spain	937.9	432.5	981.5
Sweden	974.2	599.0	1,069.2
Switzerland	825.0	526.0	1,110.5
United Kingdom	1,238.2	748.8	1,309.2
United States	1,152.7	690.7	1,163.3
		Males	
Australia	1,260.1	1,070.3	2,165.4
Austria	1,326.5	1,058.2	2,218.8
Belgium	1,492.1	1,306.0	2,857.4
Canada	1,196.7	1,090.7	2,175.4
Denmark	1,383.0	1,291.3	2,531.1
Finland	1,011.9	983.6	2,239.7
France	1,764.2	1,196.5	2,317.8
Ireland	1,281.0	1,208.0	2,528.8
Italy	1,494.7	1,224.0	2,203.7
Netherlands	1,298.8	1,259.8	2,767.6
New Zealand	1,274.2	1,145.3	2,306.4
Norway	1,113.4	1,008.2	2,281.4
Portugal	1,448.9	969.1	2,013.4
Spain	1,593.3	1,095.4	2,187.4
Sweden	946.7	854.9	1,896.1
Switzerland	1,076.0	1,018.2	2,149.8
United Kingdom	1,264.0	1,168.7	2,336.4
United States	1,327.5	1,089.9	2,031.5

SOURCES: PYLL from OECD (2000); mortality rates from WHO (2003).

NOTE: PYLL is measured as potential years of life lost per 100,000 in the relevant population. Mortality is measured as number of deaths per 100,000 in the relevant population.

Table A-4: Respiratory Disease Mortality Measures for the Countries in Our Sample

Country	PYLL	Mortality Ages 65–74	Mortality Age 75+
		Females	
Australia	142.9	136.8	472.1
Austria	89.2	56.9	377.6
Belgium	112.4	104.9	666.2
Canada	94.2	127.1	715.9
Denmark	162.3	271.7	802.3
Finland	81.4	80.0	817.4
France	77.3	59.6	653.2
Ireland	153.2	284.3	1,754.5
Italy	82.4	51.9	440.5
Netherlands	85.9	114.9	817.3
New Zealand	164.1	175.0	1,042.0
Norway	91.9	148.3	1,059.5
Portugal	170.1	104.2	794.3
Spain	91.3	73.2	682.5
Sweden	77.1	94.2	703.8
Switzerland	62.0	52.7	444.9
United Kingdom	204.6	266.2	1,605.1
United States	210.7	197.0	798.0
		Males	
Australia	176.8	256.7	950.9
Austria	123.6	174.7	659.4
Belgium	234.0	404.8	1,637.8
Canada	161.6	237.0	1,257.8
Denmark	168.3	378.1	1,334.0
Finland	172.5	279.2	1,534.8
France	169.5	183.6	1,064.9
Ireland	255.1	532.2	2,583.4
Italy	136.3	192.7	1,028.3
Netherlands	113.8	300.4	1,667.1
New Zealand	215.6	303.3	1,558.3
Norway	116.8	252.2	1,506.4
Portugal	333.5	309.6	1,407.0
Spain	254.2	306.6	1,496.7
Sweden	112.4	150.8	1,096.5
Switzerland	127.0	176.8	936.0
United Kingdom	304.2	414.0	2,148.6
United States	296.4	314.4	1,217.5

SOURCES: PYLL from OECD (2000); mortality rates from WHO (2003).

NOTE: PYLL is measured as potential years of life lost per 100,000 in the relevant population. Mortality is measured as number of deaths per 100,000 in the relevant population.

Table A-5: Explanatory Variable Measures for the Countries in Our Sample

Country	GDPPC	PHPC	HEPC	Female Smoke %	Male Smoke %	Alcohol (liters)	Female Obesity %	Male Obesity %
Australia	$16,743.99	$196.39	$1,592.34	27.0	30.2	10.5	9.1	8.2
Austria	$16,783.00	$197.43	$1,772.83	20.3	35.5	12.6	9.0	8.3
Belgium	$16,746.00	$304.47	$2,022.40	26.0	38.0	12.4	12.0	13.9
Canada	$18,555.01	$215.65	$2,170.54	26.7	29.8	9.2	13.1	13.3
Denmark	$17,096.01	$112.85	$1,839.86	42.0	47.0	11.7	7.0	8.2
Finland	$16,441.99	$190.66	$1,640.89	20.0	32.4	9.5	8.8	7.9
France	$17,655.00	$664.57	$2,155.95	19.2	37.8	16.6	6.8	6.1
Ireland	$11,388.00	$105.17	$1,029.43	29.0	31.0	10.5	9.0	12.0
Italy	$16,257.00	$447.88	$1,692.37	17.8	37.8	10.9	6.7	7.2
Netherlands	$15,921.00	$130.19	$2,103.28	31.5	42.8	9.9	8.8	6.3
New Zealand	$13,344.00	$179.31	$1,271.20	27.3	27.8	13.2	12.6	9.5
Norway	$17,514.00	$170.16	$2,011.25	33.0	36.0	5.0	5.0	6.0
Portugal	$9,598.00	$246.73	$714.33	5.8	32.4	10.1	12.6	10.3
Spain	$11,734.00	$287.41	$1,072.32	21.4	51.5	13.5	10.4	9.4
Sweden	$17,654.01	$225.86	$2,075.16	26.2	25.7	6.4	5.6	5.4
Switzerland	$21,488.01	$190.48	$2,135.27	29.0	39.0	12.9	4.7	6.0
United Kingdom	$16,055.00	$183.72	$1,525.71	29.0	31.0	9.7	15.0	13.0
United States	$22,266.01	$240.00	$2,515.00	22.8	28.4	9.5	25.1	19.9

SOURCE: OECD (2000).

Notes

1. See, for example, Newhouse (1977); Gerdtham and Jonsson (1992); and Gerdtham (1991).

2. The results were robust to the inclusion of GDP per capita (the effects of which were very imprecisely estimated) and a time trend. While the text indicated that the results included a correction for first-degree autocorrelation of the errors, the equation presented a correction for a moving-average error process. We doubt that this made much difference.

3. When conducting multivariate statistical analyses, such as regressions, the presence of either heteroskedasticity or serial correlation can cause standard errors to be estimated inaccurately. There are well-developed strategies for dealing with these problems. Or uses one of these widely accepted strategies (feasible generalized least squares) in her work.

4. In addition to this study, other authors (Murray and Lopez 1997c, 1999; Manning, Keeler, Newhouse, Sloss, and Wasserman 1991, 107–26) have looked at the impact of inactivity, which is viewed as a major contributor to obesity.

5. Strotz (1955–56) presented a nice early statement of this problem. For more recent considerations, see Becker and Mulligan (1997) or Laibson (1997).

6. Murphy and Topel (2003) have recently argued that the value of a life year gained is much higher, at $150,000–200,000 (in the United States). Cutler and McClellan (2001) have recently used a value of $100,000 per disability-free life year.

7. For an argument that ignoring quality of life understates health benefits by 30 percent, see Cutler and Richardson (1997, 262).

8. The use of medical experts has been criticized as unrepresentative of actual consumers by Cutler and Richardson (1997, 251–52).

9. Neither the WHO nor the OECD could provide cause-specific mortality data for Turkey.

10. In other words, it sets l equal to 70 in equation (1).

11. In the disease-specific mortality models, it can be argued that the optimal drug consumption measure would only measure pharmaceutical expenditures related to the specific cause of death being modeled. Such data do not exist for most countries. We did, however, check the percentage of total retail prescription

drug sales accounted for by cardiovascular and respiratory drugs in Canada, France, Italy, Spain, the United Kingdom, and the United States, using data from IMS Health's "Drug Monitor" (see OECD 2000). We found that, generally, cardiovascular drugs accounted for between 21 and 25 percent of total prescription drug sales in each country (except for the United States, where it was 19 percent), and that respiratory drugs accounted for between 8.5 and 10 percent of total sales (except for the United Kingdom, where it was 13.7 percent). These results indicated that there was likely to be only a small amount of measurement error in the drug consumption measure included in our disease-specific mortality models. Also, we would have expected any measurement error to work against finding any significant effect of drug consumption on disease-specific mortality.

12. See tables 3, 4, and 5 for descriptive statistics. The full dataset is reproduced in the appendix.

13. See, e.g., Cutler and McClellan (2001).

14. See Greene (1993, 267–70).

References

Anell, Anders and Michael Willis. 2000. International comparison of health care systems using resource profiles. *Bulletin of the World Health Organization* 78 (6): 770–78.

Babazono, Akira and Alan L. Hillman. 1994. A comparison of international health outcomes and health-care spending. *International Journal of Technology Assessment in Health Care* 10 (3): 376–81.

Becker, Gary S. and Casey B. Mulligan. 1997. The endogenous determination of time preferences. *Quarterly Journal of Economics* 112 (3): 729–58.

Bloomqvist, A. G. and R. A. L. Carter. 1997. Is health care really a luxury? *Journal of Health Economics* 16 (2): 207–29.

Bowie, C., S. Beck, G. Bevan, J. Rafferty, F. Silverton, and A. Stevens. 1997. Estimating the burden of disease in an English region. *Journal of Public Health Medicine* 19 (1): 87–92.

Cutler, David M. and Mark McClellan. 2001. Is technological change in medical care worth it? *Health Affairs* 20 (5): 11–29.

Cutler, David M. and Elizabeth Richardson. 1997. Measuring the health of the U.S. population. *Brookings papers on economic activity: Microeconomics*, 217–71.

Danzon, Patricia M. and Allison Percy. 1995. The effects of price regulation on productivity in pharmaceuticals. Unpublished paper. The Wharton School, University of Pennsylvania (July).

Frech, H. E., III and Richard D. Miller Jr. 1999. *The productivity of health care and pharmaceuticals: An international comparison.* Washington, D.C.: AEI Press.

Gerdtham, Ulf-G. 1991. *Essays on international comparisons of health care expenditure.* Linkoping Studies in Art and Sciences, no. 66. Linkoping, Sweden: Linkoping University Department of Health and Society.

Gerdtham, Ulf-G and B. Jonsson. 1992. An econometric analysis of health care expenditure: A cross section study of the OECD countries. *Journal of Health Economics* 11:63–84.

Gerdtham, Ulf-G and Michael Lothgren. 2000. On stationarity and cointegration of international health expenditure and GDP. *Journal of Health Economics* 19 (4): 461–75.

Greene, William H. 1993. *Econometric analysis.* 2nd ed. New York: Macmillan Publishing Company.

Hamilton, James D. 1994. *Time series analysis.* Princeton: Princeton University Press.

Hansen, Paul and Alan King. 1996. The determinants of health care expenditure: A cointegration approach. *Journal of Health Economics* 15 (1): 127–37.

―――. 1998. Health care expenditures and GDP: Panel data unit root tests—Comment. *Journal of Health Economics* 17 (3): 377–81.

Hill, James O. and John C. Peters. 1998. Environmental contributions to the obesity epidemic. *Science* 280 (5368): 1371–74.

Huber, P. J. 1967. The behavior of maximum likelihood estimates under non-standard conditions. In *Proceedings of the fifth Berkeley symposium on mathematical statistics and probability.* Berkeley, CA: University of California Press, 221–33.

Johannesson, Magnus. 1996. *Theory and methods of economic evaluation of health care.* Dordrecht: Kluwer Academic Publishers.

Kennedy, Peter. 1998. *A guide to econometrics.* 4th ed. Cambridge: MIT Press.

Laibson, David. 1997. Golden eggs and hyperbolic discounting. *Quarterly Journal of Economics* 112 (2): 443–77.

Lichtenberg, Frank R. 2000a. Sources of U.S. longevity increase, 1960–1997. Working paper. National Bureau of Economic Research (November).

―――. 2000b. The benefits and costs of newer drugs: Evidence from the 1996 medical expenditure panel survey. Working paper. National Bureau of Economic Research (November).

―――. 2001. Are the benefits of newer drugs worth their cost? Evidence from the 1996 MEPS. *Health Affairs* 20 (5): 241–51.

―――. 2003. Pharmaceutical innovation, mortality reduction, and economic growth. In *Measuring the gains from medical research.* Edited by Kevin M. Murphy and Robert Topel. Chicago: University of Chicago Press, 74–109.

MacDonald, Garry and Sandra Hopkins. 2002. Unit root properties of OECD health care expenditure and GDP data. *Health Economics* 11 (4): 371–76.

Manning, Willard G., Emmet B. Keeler, Joseph P. Newhouse, Elizabeth M. Sloss, and Jeffrey Wasserman. 1991. *The costs of poor health habits.* Cambridge: Harvard University Press.

McCoskey, Suzanne K. and Thomas M. Selden. 1998. Health care expenditures and GDP: Panel data unit root tests—Comment. *Journal of Health Economics* 17 (3): 369–76.

McGinnis, J. Michael and William H. Foege. 1993. Actual causes of death in the United States. *JAMA, Journal of the American Medical Association* 270 (18): 2207–13.

Miller, Richard D., Jr. and H. E. Frech III. 2000. Is there a link between pharmaceutical consumption and improved health in OECD countries? *PharmacoEconomics* 18 (Supp. 1): 33–45.

Murphy, Kevin M. and Robert Topel. 2003. The economic value of medical research. In *The value of medical research*. Edited by Kevin M. Murphy and Robert Topel. Chicago: University of Chicago Press.

Murray, Christopher J. L. and Arnab K. Acharya. 1997. Understanding DALYs. *Journal of Health Economics* 16 (6): 703–30.

Murray, Christopher J. L. and Alan D. Lopez. 1997a. Mortality by cause for eight regions of the world: Global burden of disease study. *Lancet* 349 (9061): 1269–76.

———. 1997b. Regional patterns of disability-free life expectancy and disability-adjusted life expectancy: GBD. *Lancet* 349 (9062): 1347–52.

———. 1997c. Global mortality, disability, and the contribution of risk factors: GBD. *Lancet* 349 (9063): 1436–42.

———. 1999. On the comparable quantification of health risks: Lessons from the global burden of disease study. *Epidemiology* 10 (5): 594–605.

Murray, Christopher J. L., J. Salomon, and Colin Mathers. 1999. A critical examination of summary measures of population health. Discussion Paper No. 2. Global Programme on Evidence for Health Policy, World Health Organization.

Newhouse, Joseph P. 1977. Medical-care expenditure: A cross-national survey. *Journal of Human Resources* 12 (1): 115–25.

Or, Zeynep. 2000a. Determinants of health outcomes in industrialized countries: A pooled, cross-country, time-series analysis. *OECD Economic Studies* 2000/1 (30): 53–77.

———. 2000b. Exploring the effects of health care on mortality across OECD countries. OECD labor market and social policy occasional papers, no. 46. Paris: OECD.

Organisation for Economic Co-operation and Development. 2000. *OECD health data 2000*. Paris: OECD.

———. 2003. Health at a glance: OECD indicators 2003: *Chart 8. Increasing obesity rates among the adult population in OECD countries*. OECD website. www.oecd.org/dataoecd/19/20/16361656.xls.

Peltzman, Sam. 2001. Offsetting behavior and medical breakthroughs. Working paper no. 169. George J. Stigler Center for the Study of the Economy and the State, University of Chicago.

Philipson, Tomas J. and Richard A. Posner. 1999. The long-run growth of obesity as a function of technological change. Unpublished paper. Harris School of Public Policy, University of Chicago.

Pindyck, Robert S. and Daniel L. Rubinfeld. 1998. *Econometric models and economic forecasts*. 4th ed. Boston: Irwin McGraw-Hill.

Rogers, W. H. 1993. Regression standard errors in clustered samples. *Stata Technical Bulletin* (sg17) 13:19–23. Reprinted in *Stata Technical Bulletin Reprints* 3:88–94.

Smith, Trent. 2001. Obesity and nature's thumbprint: How modern waistlines can inform economic theory. Unpublished paper. Economics Department, University of California, Santa Barbara.

Strotz, Robert H. 1955–56. Myopia and inconsistency in dynamic utility maximization. *Review of Economic Studies* 23 (3): 165–80.

Sturm, Roland. 2002. The effects of obesity, smoking and drinking on medical problems and costs. *Health Affairs* 21 (2): 245–53.

Szuba, Tadeusz J. 1986. International comparison of drug consumption: Impact of prices. *Social Science and Medicine* 22 (10): 1019–25.

White, H. 1980. A heteroskedasticity-consistent covariance matrix estimator and a direct test for heteroskedasticity. *Econometrica* 48:817–38.

Winslow, Ron and Peter Landers. 2002. Rising global obesity reflects changes in diet and lifestyles. *Wall Street Journal.* July 1.

World Health Organization. 2000. *The world health report 2000. Health systems: Improving performance.* Geneva, Switzerland: World Health Organization.

———. 2003. *WHO Mortality Database.* WHO website. www3.who.int/whosis/menu.cfm?path=whosis,whsa&language=english.

Zweifel, Peter and Matteo Ferrari. 1992. Is there a Sisyphus syndrome in health care? In *Health economics worldwide.* Edited by Peter Zweifel and H. E. Frech III. Amsterdam: Kluwer Academic Publishers, 311–30.

Index

About the Authors

Richard D. Miller Jr. is a Senior Research Analyst at the Institute for Public Research within The CNA Corporation (CNAC) in Alexandria, Virginia. He has also worked as an economist for the Bureau of Labor Statistics in Washington, D.C.

At CNAC, Mr. Miller has assessed the health-care benefits provided by the departments of Defense and Veterans Affairs, with a special focus on access to prescription drugs. He has published articles in professional journals such as *The International Journal of Health Care Finance and Economics* and *PharmacoEconomics*. He also coauthored an earlier book, *The Productivity of Health Care* and *Pharmaceuticals: An International Comparison* (AEI Press, 1999). Mr. Miller was the recipient of the Research Excellence Award for Methodology Excellence from the International Society for Pharmacoeconomics and Outcomes Research in 2001.

Mr. Miller received his doctorate in economics from the University of California, Santa Barbara in 1997.

H. E. Frech III is professor of economics at the University of California, Santa Barbara, and an adjunct professor at Sciences Po in Paris. He has been a visiting professor at Harvard University and the University of Chicago and an economist in the predecessor of the U.S. Department of Health and Human Services.

Mr. Frech has published over one hundred articles and books. He is the North American Editor of the *International Journal of the Economics of Business* and the series editor for Kluwer Academic Publishers' "Developments in Health Economics and Public Policy." His most recent books are *Competition and Monopoly in Medical Care* (AEI Press, 1996) and *The Productivity of Health Care and Pharmaceuticals: An International Comparison* (AEI Press, 1999). Mr. Frech has lectured at numerous conferences and institutions in North America and Europe.

Mr. Frech received his doctorate in economics from the University of California, Los Angeles. He is an adjunct scholar at the American Enterprise Institute.

Sam Peltzman
Ralph and Dorothy Keller
Distinguished Service Professor
of Economics
University of Chicago
Graduate School of Business

Nelson W. Polsby
Heller Professor of Political Science
Institute of Government Studies
University of California, Berkeley

George L. Priest
John M. Olin Professor of Law and
Economics
Yale Law School

Jeremy Rabkin
Professor of Government
Cornell University

Murray L. Weidenbaum
Mallinckrodt Distinguished
University Professor
Washington University

Richard J. Zeckhauser
Frank Plumpton Ramsey Professor
of Political Economy
Kennedy School of Government
Harvard University

Research Staff

Joseph Antos
Wilson H. Taylor Scholar in Health
Care and Retirement Policy

Leon Aron
Resident Scholar

Claude E. Barfield
Resident Scholar; Director, Science
and Technology Policy Studies

Roger Bate
Visiting Fellow

Walter Berns
Resident Scholar

Douglas J. Besharov
Joseph J. and Violet Jacobs
Scholar in Social Welfare Studies

Karlyn H. Bowman
Resident Fellow

John E. Calfee
Resident Scholar

Charles W. Calomiris
Arthur F. Burns Scholar in
Economics

Liz Cheney
Visiting Fellow

Lynne V. Cheney
Senior Fellow

Thomas Donnelly
Resident Fellow

Nicholas Eberstadt
Henry Wendt Scholar in Political
Economy

Eric M. Engen
Resident Scholar

Mark Falcoff
Resident Scholar

J. Michael Finger
Visiting Scholar

Gerald R. Ford
Distinguished Fellow

David Frum
Resident Fellow

Reuel Marc Gerecht
Resident Fellow

Newt Gingrich
Senior Fellow

James K. Glassman
Resident Fellow

Robert A. Goldwin
Resident Scholar

Michael S. Greve
John G. Searle Scholar

Robert W. Hahn
Resident Scholar; Director,
AEI-Brookings Joint Center
for Regulatory Studies

Kevin A. Hassett
Resident Scholar; Director, Economic
Policy Studies

Steven F. Hayward
F. K. Weyerhaeuser Fellow

Robert B. Helms
Resident Scholar; Director, Health
Policy Studies

Frederick M. Hess
Resident Scholar

R. Glenn Hubbard
Visiting Scholar

Leon R. Kass
Hertog Fellow

Jeane J. Kirkpatrick
Senior Fellow; Director, Foreign and
Defense Policy Studies

Marvin H. Kosters
Resident Scholar

Irving Kristol
Senior Fellow

Randall S. Kroszner
Visiting Scholar

Desmond Lachman
Resident Fellow

Michael A. Ledeen
Freedom Scholar

James R. Lilley
Resident Fellow

Lawrence B. Lindsey
Visiting Scholar

John R. Lott Jr.
Resident Scholar

John H. Makin
Resident Scholar; Director,
Fiscal Policy Studies

Allan H. Meltzer
Visiting Scholar

Joshua Muravchik
Resident Scholar

Charles Murray
W. H. Brady Jr. Fellow

Michael Novak
George Frederick Jewett Scholar
in Religion, Philosophy, and Public
Policy; Director, Social and Political
Studies

Norman J. Ornstein
Resident Scholar

Richard Perle
Resident Fellow

Sarath Rajapatirana
Visiting Scholar

Sally Satel
Resident Scholar

William Schneider
Resident Fellow

Daniel Shaviro
Visiting Scholar

Joel Schwartz
Visiting Scholar

J. Gregory Sidak
Resident Scholar

Radek Sikorski
Resident Fellow; Executive
Director, New Atlantic Initiative

Christina Hoff Sommers
Resident Scholar

Fred Thompson
Visiting Fellow

Peter J. Wallison
Resident Fellow

Scott Wallsten
Resident Scholar

Ben J. Wattenberg
Senior Fellow

John Yoo
Visiting Fellow

Karl Zinsmeister
J. B. Fuqua Fellow; Editor,
The American Enterprise